THE *Nourished* METABOLISM

The Balanced Guide To How
DIET, EXERCISE & STRESS
Impact Your Metabolic Health

ELIZABETH WALLING

Praise for *The Nourished Metabolism*

"As I read through this book I couldn't help but think how I wish I could have read it five years ago! I would have been spared the stress and confusion I experienced following the dietary advice of many Health and Nutrition authors. The Nourished Metabolism covers all the important aspects of health in a way that is easy to understand and follow."

>> Tiffany Pelkey from *www.thecoconutmama.com*

"After reading this book, I realized I needed to start listening to my body again. Our bodies are amazing creations and will tell us when something isn't working. Elizabeth reminded me to pay attention to how my body responds and adjust my diet as needed to get the best response."

>> Kelly Winters of *www.primallyinspired.com*

"Elizabeth provides essential information on how to heal and nourish your metabolism without fad or restrictive diets. It's a practical, doable approach to healing your metabolism for good."

>> Robin Konie of *www.thankyourbody.com*

"Whether you're just getting started on your real food journey or you've been at it for a while but feel like you could use a little help in regards to food, stress, sleep or exercise, this book will help you take your health to the next level."

>> Sylvie McCracken of *www.hollywoodhomestead.com*

Disclaimer and Copyright Information

The information in this guide is for informational purposes only. Therefore, if you wish to apply ideas contained in this book, you are taking full responsibility for your actions.

I am not a medical doctor, and the information in this book is not intended as a substitute for the medical advice of a licensed physician. The reader should regularly consult a physician in matters relating to his/her health, particularly with respect to any symptoms that may require diagnosis or medical attention.

This book is not intended to be used, nor should it be used, to diagnose or treat any medical condition. Please consult your physician for diagnosis or treatment of any medical problem. The author is not responsible for any specific health or allergy needs that may require medical supervision and is not liable for any damages or negative consequences resulting from any action by a person reading or following the information in this book.

The references provided are for informational purposes only and do not constitute endorsement of any sources.

About this Book

MY NAME IS ELIZABETH WALLING, and I've been where you are now. Whether you're just starting to research health and are confused by the mixed messages, or on the heels of yet another failed attempt at dieting, or at your wit's end wondering what in the world is safe to eat anymore, or exhausted by how complicated healthy living has become... at one time or another, I've been there, too!

I've been a health blogger since 2009, but my journey in researching health and wellness started several years earlier when I had my first child in 2004. During the past nine years, I've read countless books, articles, and blogs on eating, exercise, stress, wellness, and everything in between. And I spent a few years pretty confused by all the restrictive diet plans, extreme lifestyles, and conflicting advice.

It wasn't long before it hit me that all that restriction and obsession wasn't for me. Instead, I needed to approach eating and wellness from a balanced perspective. And I realized it had to fit into the needs of my individual body, my health, my life, and my personality.

That's why I wanted to write this book. Not only to help you find the information about health that I wish I had found at the beginning of my journey, but to let you know that it's okay to be flexible. It's okay to listen to your body. It's okay to choose what works for you. It's okay to make the plan fit *you*, instead of trying to make you fit the plan.

Well, it's not just okay—it's actually *the key* to becoming a healthy, balanced person!

So as you read this book, keep in mind that all the ideas and information you find here are meant to be flexible and adaptable to *your* life. Always listen to your body and choose what works best for you as the unique and incredible individual that you most definitely are!

» *Elizabeth*

Table of Contents

Chapter 1:
Why YOU Need a
Nourished Metabolism

ARE YOU NOURISHING YOUR METABOLISM or stressing your metabolism? The way you eat, the way you exercise—even the way you sleep—may all be working against your metabolic health. But don't be discouraged! You can change all of these things so they start working *for* your metabolism instead of against it. But first, you need to understand what your metabolism really is and what it does for you.

WHAT IS THE METABOLISM?

When you hear the word "metabolism" you probably think of burning calories. Most people do. The diet industry has hijacked the word metabolism so that people only think of it in terms of calories-in versus calories-out. But your metabolism is much more than that!

Think of your metabolism as *how your body uses energy.* But it goes way beyond just calories. Consider this: every cell in your body needs energy to function, but the health of your individual cells determines if that energy is being converted and used efficiently. Certain nutrients are needed for some cells to utilize the energy from the food you eat. If you're short on these nutrients, your cells might not be able to use energy properly. Hormones (including thyroid hormones, reproductive hormones, stress hormones, etc.) also influence how your cells process energy. How your liver processes energy can influence your thyroid health, which in turn can influence the release of stress hormones, which can affect your digestive health... It's easy to see how all of these different systems influence each other. Your metabolic health is definitely more than just how much energy you consume versus how much you use.

And *that* is how you should define your metabolism. It's not just how many calories you burn every day. Your metabolism is how every cell in your body processes and uses energy.

A NOURISHED METABOLISM VERSUS A STRESSED METABOLISM

If your metabolism isn't just about calories, then a *nourished* metabolism does more than just burn more calories—much more. In basic terms, a nourished metabolism supports healthy thyroid function, which in turn supports the quality of our moods, sleep, energy, skin, hair, and more.

When our cells get the energy they need, they are able to function at optimal levels. And when this happens, our health can finally reach an optimal state. If your cells aren't getting the energy they need to function at these levels, the metabolic rate adjusts by slowing down. Your body will also sacrifice the needs of certain systems in order to keep other more immediately important systems running.

Let's compare some basic differences between a nourished and a stressed metabolism:

NOURISHED METABOLISM

- Normal body temperature
- Level moods
- Ability to handle stress well
- Healthy hair, skin, and nails
- Excellent digestion and normal bowel movements
- Good sleep patterns

- Consistent energy
- Steady blood sugar
- Balanced hormones and a healthy sex drive

STRESSED METABOLISM

- Subnormal body temperature
- Mood swings
- Inability to handle stress
- Dry skin, dandruff, brittle nails, psoriasis, eczema, etc.
- Poor digestion, constipation, diarrhea, allergies
- Erratic sleep patterns, insomnia, trouble falling or staying asleep
- Exhaustion, alternating between wired and tired
- Blood sugar crashes
- PMS, irregular menstrual cycles, low sex drive, and other signs of hormonal imbalance

Do you have more symptoms of a nourished metabolism or a stressed metabolism?

If you experience some or all of the symptoms of a stressed metabolism—either some of the time or even most of the time—then this book was written for *you*.

HOW YOU'VE BEEN DAMAGING YOUR METABOLISM

A certain amount of metabolic decline is inevitable with age. It's just part of that thing called life. But if you're like most people, you're actively participating in accelerating the process! And you probably don't even realize you're doing it.

Everything we do—the way we eat, the way we exercise, the way we sleep, and even the way we think—contributes to **building up** or **breaking down** metabolic function. Some bad habits can do more damage than others, and some good habits can go a long way in helping you achieve outstanding metabolic health.

The trouble is that mainstream recommendations are doing a lot more harm than good. Basically, if you think you're doing everything "right" according to conventional advice or the health guru next door, you are probably putting a lot of strain on your metabolic health.

Mainstream advice is to eat a low-fat diet, avoid saturated fat, watch your salt intake, eat tons of salads, do cardio exercise for an hour or more every day... all while living the modern, high-paced lifestyle of over-packed schedules, ridiculous physique expectations, and endless amounts of stuff.

It's no wonder we're all suffering so much!

Would it surprise you to hear that you might be exercising too much and eating too little? Would it be too crazy to suggest your body probably needs more saturated fat and more salt? If you think I'm insane for even suggesting these things, keep reading. There's sound science to back it all up.

If you want to change your health, you have to change your habits. Some changes are going to be easy-peasy. Others may feel like nails on a chalkboard, especially if you are fighting bad health dogma and lifelong habits.

But they say if you want different results, you have to stop trying the same thing over and over. So we're going to try something different. Instead of starving your body, we're going to nourish your metabolism.

HOW TO NOURISH YOUR METABOLISM

By the end of this book, you're going to know what you've been doing right and what you've been doing wrong—and it may not be what you think! I like to keep things simple. Small adjustments really do add up over time, so you won't hear me recommending anything like a two-week detox or an extreme pantry clean out. You don't need to throw away all the food in your cupboards or drink green juices for a month just to get healthy. In fact, that's the kind of behavior you need to trash if you want to live nourished!

Instead, you're going to see how the different areas of your life are affecting your metabolism. Where you need the most help depends on your current diet, lifestyle, and the state of your metabolic health. But the important part is to see how it all fits together.

Diet, exercise, and stress are all inexplicably linked together. They all influence each other, and they all affect your metabolic state. If you're doing everything right on one side, you can effectually cancel out your positive behavior by doing everything wrong on the other side! And that's exactly why so many people feel like they're going in circles trying to get healthy—always moving but never really getting anywhere.

So you're going to learn how to keep it all in balance. In the chapters ahead, you'll find simple tips and tweaks that you can start using right away. No fear-mongering, no pressure to be perfect, and no extreme lifestyle overhauls in 30 days. None of that here. We're here to make real, positive, *lasting* changes. Because that's the only kind of change that really counts.

HERE'S WHAT YOU'RE GOING TO LEARN:

- We'll take a look at the big one: stress. I'll be busting popular myths and misconceptions about what stress is and how it affects your body. We'll look at all different types of stress and how to reduce or eliminate them.

- We'll cover how to eat a balanced diet that gives your body the energy and nutrients it needs to function at its best. We're going to bust through fad diets, forget about dietary dogma, and look at the real basics of eating well for a nourished metabolism. You'll also learn common eating mistakes that could be stressing your metabolism and preventing it from going to the next level.

- Next, you'll learn whether your exercise and sleep habits are helping or hurting your metabolism. Chances are, you have the wrong ideas about exercise! And even more importantly, you may not be getting the sleep you need to nourish your metabolic health.

MY JOURNEY TO A NOURISHED METABOLISM

Are you tired of having a stressed metabolism? I've been there! And I'm living proof that habits can be changed, and a stressed metabolism can become a nourished one.

A few years ago, I showed every sign of having a stressed metabolism. I had trouble falling asleep every night, and then I'd wake up in the wee hours of the morning and couldn't fall back asleep for hours. I was exhausted all day, my moods were erratic, and I had no less than two weeks of crippling PMS symptoms every month. I was hungry every 30 minutes because my blood sugar was completely out of whack, and my skin somehow managed to be really dry and really oily all at the same time.

Not to mention, my hands and feet were often cold—even in the summer. And my ability to handle stress of any kind? Non-existent. Not good when you're a mom of two toddlers!

To put it simply, life was losing its luster. And I was only in my early twenties! I knew this was no way to live. There had to be a way to feel healthy, to *be* healthy. And so, being the bookworm that I am, I started reading. And reading. And reading. I read book after book on diet, exercise, stress, mental health, and anything else I could get my hands on.

It was a lot of information (probably too much), and a lot of it was conflicting. I realized I was going to have to sift through fact and fiction to figure out what actually works in the real world. And even more importantly, what would work for *my* body and lifestyle.

Right away, I realized most health books were missing something. They had some pieces right, but they would neglect other important factors. Some put too much focus on eating the perfect diet and creating a web of rigid rules for every meal. Others emphasized exercise (and typically the wrong kind, as I later discovered), taking a bunch of supplements, and drinking lots of water. Still others looked mostly at the mental side of things: how the way we think affects our health and wellness.

But few authors wrote about how all of these are connected. What we eat can affect how we think. And what we think can affect how we eat. How we exercise can influence our sleeping patterns, and sleeping well can help give us the energy we need to be active. Supplements can help, but they can also do more harm than good.

Unfortunately, I was weaving my way in and out of this web of occasionally helpful and sometimes really confusing information all on my own. I did a lot of wrong things on my road to good health. So many times it was two steps forward and one step back. I had good months and bad months; but after a few years, I finally had it nailed.

Today, I can finally sleep a good eight to nine hours every night. I can handle a heck of a lot more stress than I used to—which is a good thing, because life has thrown me some curveballs! My energy levels are pretty consistent, and I no longer need an afternoon nap just to make it through the day. My hands and feet are rarely cold, except maybe on the most bitterly cold of winter days. And my skin and hair have never looked better, in spite of the fact that I've aged a few years since.

I still have good days and bad days, of course—a nourished metabolism doesn't make you superhuman! But typically, the good days outnumber the bad; and the lows are never as low as they used to be. And even more, I know the signs of a stressed metabolism; and I have the tools I need to recognize them and prevent my health from slipping back downhill.

And that, to me, is called a nourished life.

Chapter 2:
The Metabolism Killer

STRESS IS OFTEN MISLABELED AND MISUNDERSTOOD. Most people think of stress as being "stressed out" emotionally, but it can be caused by a variety of events—many of which aren't emotional at all! There are a lot of misconceptions about what stress really is and how it impacts our health. But understanding stress and how it affects your metabolism is one of the most important things you can do for your health.

WHAT IS STRESS?

Physiologically, stress could be considered any event that triggers a marked response by the adrenal glands. In basic terms, this response is the release of the stress hormones like adrenaline and cortisol. It's the body's natural reaction to *any* stressor. **Your body doesn't distinguish between different kinds of stress. It responds to every stress in the same way.**

For occasional stressors, stress hormones can provide a burst of benefits like increased energy, heightened reflexes, and a higher threshold for pain. But with chronic stress—which is the norm in our society—stress hormone levels can remain unnaturally high and will eventually lead to damaging side effects.

Adrenaline and cortisol are not meant to be chronically high; and when they are, they take their toll on the body.

THE (FALSE) FEEL-GOOD PHASE

The problem is this: stress hormones can make you feel good... in the short-term. They can even reduce inflammation and seemingly solve a variety of health issues... again, in the short-term. That's why pretty much every diet under the sun has a following of folks who experienced weight-loss, high levels of energy, euphoria, and the disappearance of issues like skin inflammation, digestive problems, etc. I call this the False Feel-Good Phase.

This can look really confusing from the outside, when you see people experiencing similar benefits on diets that appear to be total opposites: low-fat and high-fat, vegan and all-meat, high-starch and low-carb. But these benefits are almost always *short-term*. For pretty much every diet under the sun, there is an equal following who has faithfully followed the rules only to experience a sudden decline in their results and their health as the weeks or months wear on.

Why? **Because the diets themselves trigger the stress response.** Your body perceives these diets as stressors because they cause energy deprivation, in one form or another, which your body only knows as famine. And a famine is definitely a stress!

The initial surge of stress hormones triggered by a restrictive diet can make you feel like you're on top of the world. The new diet (whatever it is) seems effortless to follow, you have oodles of energy, and everything in life just looks peachy.

But the positive effects of stress hormones are *temporary*. They are meant to be. They are nature's way of supporting you through a fight-or-flight situation—you know, like getting chased by a lion!

Stress hormones break down proteins from your muscles and bones; and over time, your lean body tissues deteriorate. They also deny energy to lesser systems in the body—the kind that aren't important when you're trying to outrun that lion—like digestive function and mood health. That's why poor digestion and low moods are some of the earliest symptoms of chronically high stress hormones.

And this doesn't just happen with diets. The False Feel-Good

Phase can occur when you start a new vigorous workout routine, or even when you take on a huge project at work. In the beginning, there is plenty of motivation and energy to go around; but after a while, you suddenly feel drained, your sleep suffers, and your mental function isn't at its best.

These are all side effects of chronically high stress hormones. Here are some other symptoms you might experience:

- Poor thyroid function
- Blood sugar swings
- Loss of lean body tissue like muscle and bone mass
- Mood swings and depression
- High blood pressure
- Sleep problems
- Inflammatory skin conditions like eczema
- Susceptibility to illness and infection
- Weight gain, particularly in the abdominal region

As time passes, chronically high stress hormones contribute to further degeneration. This is when the risk for serious problems like cancer, heart disease, and dementia increases. Yes, high stress hormones are just the gift that keeps on giving.

WHAT CAUSES STRESS? IT'S NOT ALWAYS WHAT YOU THINK

Understanding what constitutes stress is one of the most

important keys to dealing with it. Otherwise, you could very well be letting untold sources of stress slip through your fingers without notice. Here is a breakdown of common stressors:

EMOTIONAL AND PSYCHOLOGICAL STRESS. This is what we normally think of as stress. This includes an unhappy work situation, dysfunctional relationships, negative thought patterns, or loss of a loved one—but it can also be more subtle. Any situation that drains you mentally and emotionally, day in and day out, is a source of stress. We all have times of stress at work and in our relationships, but it becomes a problem when the stress is part of your everyday life without end in sight. That's a sign that something needs to change.

LACK OF SLEEP, RELAXATION, AND DOWNTIME. This is all too common in our society where many people sacrifice sleep and downtime in order to get more done. If you regularly work late into the night—whether you're preparing a presentation or hand-sewing Halloween costumes for the kids—stress is going to be a problem.

ALLERGIES. Allergens in food or in your environment can cause stress; and stress can, in turn, trigger allergic reactions. This results in a vicious cycle which is sure to wear you down. Allergies can come from a variety of sources, and not always the obvious ones. You may have hay fever or pet allergies, or you could just have a gluten allergy that's been flying under your radar for years. I don't believe in becoming obsessed with finding food allergies (obsession is really just another form of stress!), but it is something to consider.

POOR EATING HABITS AND DIET. A healthy, balanced diet is the foundation of metabolic health. Skipping meals, dieting, or cutting out food groups can all be significant stressors. Unfortunately, these habits are all too common in our culture—many times they are even encouraged! Far too many people overload on caffeine during the day to avoid eating, only to binge on a bunch of empty calories before bed. It's another vicious cycle that stresses the body on so many levels.

EXCESSIVE EXERCISE. Staying active is an important part of a healthy lifestyle; but the mantra of "exercise more" is repeated so often, people tend to think more is *always* better. This is not necessarily true. Over-exercising is just as bad as not exercising at all, if not worse, especially if you have a stressed metabolism. Exercise should be incorporated into a healthy lifestyle, but exercise in no way makes up for unhealthy living. In fact, exercising too much when your metabolic health is poor can actually make things even worse.

PHYSICAL STRESSORS. Whether it's a common cold or a sports injury, illness and physical trauma are stressors. Recurring infections, chronic pain, or repeat injuries are especially stressful, and they are also signs of a stressed metabolism. Surgery can also be considered a physical trauma, which is why it's important to take extra care of yourself while recovering from surgery or injury.

TOXIN EXPOSURE. This includes substances like refined foods, chemical food additives (such as MSG), nicotine, airborne pollution, chemicals found in household cleaners, toxins in our water supply, and the host of other chemicals and toxins we encounter every day. These chemicals can affect our bodies at a cellular level, which can impact our metabolic health. It's impossible to avoid all toxins in modern society, but there are certainly some simple steps you can take to dramatically reduce your exposure to these substances.

NOT ENOUGH SUNLIGHT. Being indoors and away from natural light is a stressor on the body. This is partly why winter months often trigger depression, moodiness, lethargy, and other symptoms of Seasonal Affective Disorder (SAD). Studies have linked SAD with low thyroid function (which means low metabolic function), while too much melatonin (a biochemical released when you're in darkness) has been linked to high cortisol levels and depression. If you spend most of the daytime indoors and out of natural light, you're essentially putting your body through the same type of stress—effectively making SAD last all year long! You are also limiting your body's natural production of vitamin D, which requires sunlight.

The above list is meant to be used as a resource for identifying the top sources of stress in your life. It's not possible to avoid every single one of these stressors—in fact, you are sure to encounter many of them throughout your life.

But whenever possible, make positive changes in order to reduce the number or intensity of stressors you experience. If you're experiencing unavoidable stress in one area, make up for it by trying to reduce stress in another way. Aim for the easy changes first, so you can start moving in a positive direction right away. It can have a substantial impact on your physical and emotional health.

HOW TO LIMIT STRESS

Once you've identified the tops sources of stress in your life, it's time to take action by making those positive habit shifts. Most people are amazed at the improvement they see in their health after making just a few small but significant changes in how they deal with stress.

Below are a few quick suggestions for getting started coping with the different stressors in your life. I'll get into several of them in much greater detail in later chapters.

REDUCE EMOTIONAL AND PSYCHOLOGICAL STRESS. The impact of emotional stress cannot be underestimated, but this type of stress is often overlooked because it's not easy to change it. A difficult living situation, an unhealthy relationship, or a stressful job could be a source of major stress that is wearing down your health. This doesn't necessarily mean you have to move, become a hermit, or quit your job; but it's important to look for ways to improve your situation in whatever way you can.

Although it appears insignificant on the surface, negative thought patterns have a way of chipping away at our quality of life by compounding our stress. Because we can't expect our circumstances and relationships to always go our way, we need to learn to cope with negative situations in a positive way. Establishing healthy patterns of enjoying the moment, reframing negative thoughts, and learning to forgive can have a positive effect on your health.

If you're dealing with other stressors like depression, anxiety, or the loss of a loved one, you may want to seek counseling or join a support group that can offer you help.

PRIORITIZE QUALITY SLEEP AND DOWNTIME. The impact sleep can have on your life is well documented. Getting *at least* seven hours every night can help regulate your stress hormone levels, improve your energy, and brighten your mood.

And just as important as sleep is *downtime*. It may take some rearranging if your schedule is packed with activities, but it's vital for your health to take time each day to relax and unwind. Taking a day off now and then to free yourself from that mile-long to-do list is restorative as well. And by all means, if you can take a vacation and get away from it all—do it!

IMPROVE YOUR EATING HABITS AND THE QUALITY OF YOUR FOOD. It can't be emphasized enough: *food is the foundation of your health*. A balanced diet of quality food is a must. Avoid eating way too much processed food, skipping meals or under-eating. Your body needs real food to rebuild and nourish your metabolism.

AVOID ALLERGENS. If you have allergies, these can trigger a stress response in the body. Do your best to identify and avoid allergens so you can make better food choices. On the upside, as your metabolic health improves, you may notice a decrease in the severity of your allergic reactions (which are, in part, a stress response of their own). This is because a nourished metabolism has a healthy immune response.

Many people notice that once they are metabolically healthy, they can tolerate substances that previously caused reactions. I personally developed a nasty reaction to cashews after my first pregnancy. Several years later after learning healthy habits, I can now eat cashews with no issues whatsoever! (Note: This is not a license to eat anything you're allergic to; be wise and consult a doctor first.)

EXERCISE THE SMART AND SENSIBLE WAY. Being active provides metabolic benefits, but it's important not to overdo it if you're otherwise stressed. Emphasize activities like strength training, yoga, walking, and swimming. Avoid overtraining or doing too much cardio (aerobic) exercise, which tends to be the most stressful kind.

REDUCE PHYSICAL STRESSORS. If you get sick, injured, or have to deal with chronic pain, try to get the rest and care you need so you can reduce the stress these cause on your body. Allow your body time to heal, or in the case of chronic pain, look for ways to treat the pain or the underlying cause.

REDUCE YOUR EXPOSURE TO TOXINS. Most of us can't completely eliminate toxins from our lives, but we can take measures to greatly reduce the amount of toxins our bodies must deal with every day. Filter your water, use natural beauty and cleaning products, eat organic foods, avoid chemical food additives, and enjoy fresh air as much as you can.

GET PLENTY OF NATURAL LIGHT EXPOSURE. Try to spend more time outdoors in natural light. Aim for at least 20 minutes a day, if possible. Develop hobbies that encourage you to be outdoors during the day: hiking, gardening, walking, biking, birdwatching, etc.

If you have to live with long winters or a rainy climate, it can help to try light therapy to mimic exposure to natural sunlight. Expensive light boxes aren't really necessary. A simple, high-wattage incandescent bulb can be enough to mimic the sun's warm light. Try 15-20 minutes in the morning when you first wake up to help regulate your circadian rhythms. But getting outdoors in the natural light is always preferable.

Stress may come at you from every corner; but through small and consistent changes, you can avoid some potential stressors and learn to cope with stress you can't avoid. When you start building healthy habits, you'll reduce the overall stress load on your metabolism. This sets up a snowball effect of positive changes in your metabolic function, which will not only help your body cope with stress in the future, but will reward you with more vibrant health along the way.

Chapter 3:
Dieting: The Ultimate
Metabolic Stressor

HOW MANY TIMES HAVE YOU PICKED UP a new diet book in hopes that it would finally be the answer you've been looking for? And how many times did you find yourself back at square one: looking for another new diet book just a few months later?

In fact, if you're like most people, you've probably tried following several if not dozens of different diets. You've done the cleanses and the jump-starts and the 21-day detoxes and everything in between. How do I know? Because I've done it all too! But every diet ended in with the same result: failure. Sometimes I'd lose some weight just to gain it back later.

Sometimes I'd have a few symptoms get better only to have a whole new set of symptoms appear!

You might be saying to yourself, "But it's my own fault! I didn't follow the plan. If I had more willpower, I could have stuck with the meal plan and stopped eating all those bad foods. Then I'd be healthy and thin. I just couldn't follow the plan."

In fact, I bet you've said this to yourself every time you've jumped on another diet bandwagon. Every time you convince yourself *this* diet will change everything. *This* diet will solve your health issues. And *this* diet will help you get thin.

It hasn't worked yet, has it? But we repeat the same pattern over and over again, somehow expecting different results.

Well, now is the time for *real* change. It's not a new diet plan or exercise routine you need to follow. You don't need a new plan; you need a new *approach*. You have to approach diet and exercise in a way you never have before.

Jumping from diet to diet in hopes of achieving lasting positive change is not the solution. In fact, *it's distracting you from the solution*. The real solution is slowing down and becoming aware of what your body really needs. And if you take time to think about it, you know your body doesn't need another fad diet or boot camp. It doesn't need another tortured experience of deprivation and physical strain.

You've got to let go of the part of you that keeps saying, "Just one more diet. Just let me go on the grapefruit diet, lose those last ten pounds, and *then* I can take care of myself."

You need to take care of yourself *now*. Not tomorrow or next month. Not ten pounds from now. The longer you delay nourishing your metabolism, the more likely you'll face all those unpleasant side effects of a stressed metabolism, and the more likely they'll just continue to get worse over time.

Do you really want to look back in a year—or five or ten years—and wonder why you wasted all that time suffering?

The truth is, you can start turning your health around now and reap the benefits of a nourished metabolism. But you do have to make a choice. You have to choose to give up on fad diets and magic pills. You have to choose to start living well and nourishing yourself today, one step at a time. Otherwise you're choosing to deal with side effects like low energy, PMS, thinning hair, poor libido, cold hands and feet, constipation, chronic back pain, and all that good stuff.

I'm sorry I can't give you a magic pill. Trust me, I've looked for it but never found it. And looking for a quick fix just made me more miserable because it never addressed the *real* issues. It just swept them under the rug so they could rear their ugly heads again later. And they just got uglier until I finally realized that genuinely nourishing myself was the *only* way to achieve real health and wellness.

BUSTING THE DIET MYTH

So no, I'm not going to tell you what you want to hear. I'm not going to make promises about melting fat away in your sleep or finally wearing that tiny bikini lurking in the back of your closet. If you're reading this book, then you may be interested in losing some weight; but right now I want to focus on the subject that's often left to the wayside when weight loss is on the mind: your health.

Diet gurus are smart: most of them realize we don't want to knowingly sacrifice our health in order to lose weight, so they promote their diets as both effective *and* healthy. In fact, they make it seem like weight loss and health go hand in hand. "Lose weight, get healthy" is the message. But more often than not, this is just a marketing ploy that doesn't hold water in the real world.

This is partially because the diet industry assumes the body can be reduced down to calories in versus calories out. It's all about numbers. When you eat this much or weigh that much, you're automatically healthy. But as we've been discussing, the body is really an incredibly complex system of cells, energy, hormones, biochemicals, reactions, and instincts. You can't go on a diet without affecting all of these systems.

Your body is constantly regulating temperature, acidity, energy conversion, and a variety of other factors to make sure it's functioning at the best it can at any given moment.

What you're eating, thinking, and doing has a direct impact on this process.

Dieting is like dropping a bomb into this complex structure and hoping nothing will go wrong. The most common bomb is low-calorie dieting—in its many, many forms—which is the idea that you can starve the fat off your body (either quickly or slowly). The very premise of this theory is flawed, because your body is made to fight against starvation by down-regulating your metabolism. It's your body's natural response to cope with times when the food supply is restricted—even when *you're* the one restricting it.

Here's a quick example of ways your body will cope with dieting:

- **REDUCING THE METABOLISM BY TURNING DOWN THYROID FUNCTION.** Long-term dieting or frequent yo-yo dieting can lead to some heavy thyroid damage. Many dieters have the telltale low basal temperature as evidence of low thyroid function.

- **STIMULATING THE ADRENAL GLANDS** to release adrenaline and cortisol to cope with this "famine" period (because that's what a lack of food means to your body). These stress hormones are meant to keep your vital organs functioning during times of stress. But chronic dieting keeps these stress hormones unnaturally high for long periods of time, which leads to symptoms of a stressed metabolism.

- **BREAKING DOWN LEAN TISSUE MASS.** High stress hormones and a lack of energy from food triggers the body to start breaking down lean body mass like muscle, bone, and organ tissue to supply the body with what it needs. Muscle burns fat, so when muscle is broken down, you actually end up burning *less* fat than before you started dieting!

- **PRIORITIZING CERTAIN FUNCTIONS OVER OTHERS.** With a limited amount of food coming in, the body gets choosy with how it's spending energy. Regulating moods, for instance, might take a low priority because feeling happy and balanced isn't as important as basic survival during a time of famine. Mood problems, thinning hair, sleep disturbances, and skin problems are among the first to show up as the metabolism copes with dieting.

Thyroid health is at the center of metabolic function, and eating enough food is very important for maintaining a healthy thyroid. To quote Julia Ross in her book, *The Mood Cure*:

Getting adequate calories and avoiding low-cal dieting is essential for keeping the thyroid gland turned on or for turning it up once it's been turned down. According to the World Health Organization, **that means approximately 2,100 calories or more per day for females and 2,300 for males.** *[my emphasis in bold]*

So while we may work tirelessly to end starvation in third-world countries, in Western society, we are starving ourselves *on purpose*. And our metabolic health is suffering as a consequence.

WHY DIETING IS SO DIFFICULT

Most of us are conditioned to automatically believe eating less and exercising more will lead to good health. But many times, the opposite is true. In fact, it's not unusual for people to trace their health problems back to their first diets.

Have you ever wondered why it's so hard to diet and why it doesn't always work? Why do we have to force ourselves to cut calories or carbs to lose weight? These are the questions we need to be asking, because we keep trying to use the same ineffective methods over and over again. But with modern society pounding the same message into our heads every day, it can be difficult to think outside of the diet-and-exercise box.

Most doctors, physical trainers, nutritionists, and dieticians offer the same solution. It's like the mantra of the modern age: "You're overweight. You must be eating too much. You must not be active enough. Everything will fix itself once you start eating less and exercising more."

It doesn't help that this often works, but only in the short term. In fact, the first couple of diets we ever go on are often our most successful. I remember on my first diet (at the tender age of thirteen), it was almost painless to cut back on eating and exercise more; and the weight came off almost effortlessly. Just like that, I was hooked.

Now it's ingrained in our heads: eating less and exercising more works. We've seen it work. If we're gaining weight again, it's *our* problem. We must not have enough willpower, enough determination, enough drive. If we could only stick with the plan, we'd enjoy that same success again. We'd be able to lose weight and keep it off forever.

If only we could stick to the plan.

Ever wonder why sticking to the plan is so hard? Most people will say it's a matter of willpower, implying that you're just too lazy or you just don't care enough to follow the plan. And on the surface, this can appear to be true.

But internally, there's a different story going on. You know that frustrated feeling that your body is fighting you every step of the way while you're dieting? Well, you're right! To be more accurate, *you're* fighting with your body; and your body is fighting back with all it's got. Why? It's a natural biological response. **This is the way your body responds to dieting.**

Doesn't it make sense? Our bodies are designed to cope with the elements. Traditionally, the most common stressors your body encountered were things like famine and cold. How does it cope when faced with these situations? **By releasing stress hormones and storing fat.**

It's an incredibly effective model. When you start dieting, the appetite goes up and so does fat storage. At the same time, your energy levels go down so you're not in the mood to hop on the treadmill. Every single biochemical reaction in your body is rigged to save every ounce of fat it can.

This is why diets ultimately fail. Every diet that forces your body to do the opposite of what it's striving for will result in an even more exaggerated response. If you diet "harder," your body will fight back even harder. This is why it's not uncommon to regain weight lost during a diet, plus a little extra. The body pads on a little more because it's biochemically convinced this is what's necessary for survival.

The key is telling your body there won't be any more famines.

How can you convince the body it's not in the midst of a

terrible famine or traumatic stress? You have to nourish yourself! This means eating nutritious foods when you're hungry, and taking care of your body with the right exercise and quality sleep. Stop viewing your body as the enemy. Stop working against your body's natural mechanisms. Instead, work *with* your body by listening to your biofeedback and responding with what it needs.

DIETS DON'T ACTUALLY WORK

There are multitudes of dieters that could tell you how diets don't work in the long run. But you may be surprised to hear that research actually backs up these claims.

- Researchers at UCLA looked at the results of 31 long-term studies on dieting. These studies provided unique information about the effectiveness of dieting, because they followed up with dieters after two to five years (most dieting studies follow up for only one year or less). They found that the average dieter can lose about five to ten percent of their body weight within the first six months of dieting. But five years later, as many as two-thirds of dieters have regained *more* weight than they lost.

- Another study at the University of Melbourne looked at the effect of dieting on 100 overweight men and women. Participants lost weight after being on a strict diet for the first eight weeks and were then counseled about healthy eating habits so they could maintain their weight loss.

But most participants regained the weight they lost and reported being more hungry and obsessed with food than before the diet. Starting to sound familiar?

- A Pennsylvania State University study followed a group of women for six years to see if dieting predicted weight change over time. Researchers found that women who reported dieting at the beginning of the study were heavier and gained more weight over the course of the study than non-dieters.

NOTE: If you see a study touting a successful weight loss diet, take it with a grain of salt. Most diet studies follow participants for only a few weeks or months. Studies that follow up with dieters after a few years reveal that the majority of dieters regain what they lost—and sometimes even more.

THE DANGERS OF DIETING

Putting yourself through another diet isn't just ineffective in the long run. It can also be downright unhealthy. There is an entire body of research that shows how dieting leads to metabolic disorders that actually do more harm to your health than just being overweight!

Say what? It sounds crazy, I know. We're constantly told that carrying a few extra pounds is dangerous to our health, but science says otherwise. The metabolic effects of dieting are a serious concern; but in our diet-loving society, these problems are often swept under the rug in favor of the latest eating plan and exercise video.

The evidence strongly indicates that dieting affects far more than just your body fat levels: dieting affects you—and can harm you—on a metabolic level. Here are just a few of the ways dieting can be detrimental to your long-term health:

- Research shows that weight fluctuations are actually *more* dangerous than just carrying excess weight. A history of weight cycling (yo-yo dieting) is strongly associated with an increased risk for developing metabolic conditions like heart disease as well as an increased mortality rate. This is independent of weight, so it applies whether you're a dieter who is skinny or one who's heavy.

- One study showed that obese women who diet are far more likely to have high blood pressure than obese women who do not have a history of dieting. Again, the act of dieting itself appears more damaging than just carrying some extra weight.

- Weight loss that comes through dieting (especially extreme dieting) always risks losing lean body tissue in addition to fat. This robs your muscles, bones, and organs of the material they need to function properly. While some diets increase this risk more than others, it is a risk with *all* diets that have you restricting calories, which is most diets in one form or another.

- Our kids pick up on our obsessions with weight and our eating habits. Whether we realize it or not, we often project our own insecurities about weight and dieting onto our kids. It's hard not to do. But research shows that parents who impose restrictive eating habits only encourage further weight gain in their children. If you ask me, stopping this vicious cycle in its tracks is reason enough to swear off dieting forever.

- Dieting distorts our natural relationship with hunger and food. When food is considered "good" or "bad," eating becomes a moral issue rather than an act of nourishment. When we deny our hunger, we forget how to eat for natural reasons. Instead, we develop habits of emotional eating and experience guilt or shame when we eat the "wrong" food. Basically, we forget how to eat! This leads to obsessive thought patterns and a distorted body image, both of which are a damaging source of stress that no one needs.

Though the dangers of dieting are all too real, millions of people ignore these risks every day in order to reach a magical number on the scale. But extreme diets and obsessive behavior are not part of living a nourished life. They only get in the way of your efforts to improve your metabolic health.

DITCH THE DIETS FOR GOOD

If all of this sounds discouraging, don't lose hope! Realistic weight loss is possible, but *first* you have to establish healthy living habits and healthy attitudes about food.

Don't play the game of dieting now and getting healthy later because more often than not, later never really comes; and you just get stuck in an endless loop of yo-yo dieting. Instead, embrace a lifestyle that brings you long-term success and truly nourishes your body from the inside out. It's time to end your struggle with your body and ditch the diets for good.

Chapter 4:
Digestion: The Energy
Gateway

METABOLIC ENERGY HINGES ENTIRELY ON DIGESTION. If you can't digest food and fully break down its nutrients, then even the best food choices are going to have a limited impact on your health, because your metabolism isn't getting the energy and nutrients it needs for optimal function.

When it comes to healing yourself from the inside out, taking care of your gut health should make the top of your priority list. With so much emphasis put on the health of the heart, brain, liver, and lungs, it's easy to forget that the gut is where many health problems begin. Achieving a healthy digestive system is a key step toward improving health in every system in the body.

Today, many people tend to think digestive upsets like heartburn, acid reflux, IBS (irritable bowel syndrome), stomach pains, and constipation are normal, everyday occurrences. In fact, we have entire aisles at the store dedicated solely to medications designed to treat these symptoms. And yes, they are *symptoms*—signs of poor gut health. But when we focus solely on treating the symptoms, we ignore the larger issue and damage our metabolic health as a result.

Digestive problems have reached almost epidemic proportions, especially for the youngest generation. Even young babies are developing acid reflux and leaky gut syndrome. This is because gut flora are established in utero, at childbirth, and also during the early months of breastfeeding. If the mother has an imbalance of bacteria in *her* gut, this is passed on to her baby.

And that's just the beginning. Once you begin with poor gut function, it's a snowball effect from there. Poor digestion leads to poor energy, which leads to poor thyroid function. Then you have an environment where toxic bacteria are able to thrive in your gut, which in turn leads to—you guessed it—even more damage to the digestive system.

If the cycle continues, your body gets less and less of the energy and nutrients it needs as your digestive system struggles with bacterial imbalances and inflammation. Food allergies can develop, as well as seemingly unrelated conditions like skin disorders, autoimmune conditions, and mood problems. But all of these symptoms are very much related to one another. *It all started in your gut.*

GUT HEALTH 101

What does the gut really do? We know what the heart does, we know what the lungs do. Some of us would even venture to say we have a good grasp on what the liver and kidneys do. But what about our gut? We know it's responsible for digesting food, but in reality the gut handles a lot more than we think.

- The gut is like an intricate ecosystem populated with an incredible amount of living beings: tiny microorganisms which play a key role in keeping you healthy. Your body relies on this population of beneficial bacteria to assimilate valuable nutrients and to defend itself against toxins and pathogenic bacteria.

- About 70-80% of your immune system in based in your gut. A healthy gut can put up an awesome fight against invading bacteria and viruses. On the same note, a weak gut makes you vulnerable to a myriad of illnesses and conditions, because a compromised immune system can lead to inflammatory and autoimmune conditions.

- You probably know the saying "follow your gut feeling." Well, in a way you really *can* think with your gut!

Containing more nerve cells and neurotransmitters than your nervous system, the gut has been referred to as a second brain. And what goes on in there is just as important as what's going on in your brain.

HOW THE BAD GUYS TOOK OVER

Once upon a time, no one had to put much thought into gut health. When babies were born and breastfed, they inherited their mother's balanced gut bacteria. With a lifestyle that supported metabolic health (i.e. nutritious food and healthy living), their bodies were able to maintain proper balance in their digestive systems to fight inflammation and keep everything running smoothly.

Unfortunately, the path to excellent digestive health is not so easy today. Many of us start off life with compromised gut health, and it just gets worse from there. Chemical additives, antibiotics, and indigestible material lurk in most of the foods we eat; and key nutrients that support gut health are missing from the modern diet. Stress increases inflammation, which just compounds these problems.

Under these conditions, bad bacteria and fungi (like candida, or yeast) flourish. They feed on the indigestible material we consume, and our guts have become too weak to fight them off. These pathogens produce toxins that leak through our weakened gut walls and move on to poison the rest of our body. The cycle continues as the pathogens gain more power in our digestive systems. It seems like a fight we can't win, but we have more control over our gut health than it seems.

So, how do you restore your gut health? There are six important keys to healing your gut and improving your digestion:

1. NOURISH YOUR METABOLISM.

It may seem redundant to come back to this, but it's important to put the horse before the cart. If you only do the "right" things to help your gut, but don't work on your overall metabolic health, you're just going to go in circles and never see real progress.

A healthy metabolism supports your gut. When your metabolic health is top-notch, your body temperature is normal; inflammation is low; and your immune system is strong. These all help to keep pathogenic bacteria in check so they don't wreak havoc on your digestion and the integrity of your gut.

So while the rest of the steps we'll talk about are important, keep in mind that a nourished metabolism is still your foundation for good health. Without it, you'll only see minimal results.

2. ADDRESS THE STRESS.

While this goes right along with nourishing your metabolism, lowering stress levels is so important it warrants an extra mention. Stress, from whatever source, restricts blood flow to the digestive system. This impairs proper digestion and weakens the integrity of the gut lining over time, which can increase the uptake of toxins from the gut. **Reducing stress is paramount for healing your gut and improving digestion.**

3. AVOID FOODS AND SUBSTANCES THAT IRRITATE YOUR GUT.

Did you know that many of the foods you eat and supplements you take may be irritating your gut and feeding pathogens in your digestive system?

Here are some common problems in the modern diet that can lead to gut irritation:

Too much fiber. Most people are told more fiber is better—stock up on leafy greens, beans, legumes, and whole grains. And if that isn't enough, pile on the wheat germ and psyllium husk. But there is such a thing as too much fiber.

Fiber is indigestible. That's why it's said to add "bulk" to your diet—your body cannot digest it, so it sticks around in the digestive tract. And because of this, fiber provides no metabolic energy whatsoever. It is essentially an empty food.

But fiber can actually be even worse than empty—fiber can prevent the absorption of important minerals like zinc, magnesium, and calcium. There is also evidence that certain fibers can interfere with protein absorption.

A common misconception is that fiber feeds "good" bacteria

exclusively. The truth is, all kinds of bacteria feed on fiber. So if you already have a bacterial imbalance in your gut, eating too much fiber could make it worse.

Keep in mind, that this doesn't mean that you shouldn't consume *any* fiber. Fiber does provide some unique benefits as well. For instance, fiber helps beneficial bacteria produce short-chain fatty acids in the gut, which are associated with anti-inflammatory benefits.

So it's important to keep a balanced view of fiber in mind. In particular, take note of how your digestion is affected by certain fiber-rich foods. Grains, beans, and nuts may be particularly irritating to someone with an extremely sensitive gut, while fresh fruit can be especially healing to others. Listen to your body and don't eat too much of the foods that seem to cause a lot of gas, bloating, or stomach pain.

Carrageenan. Carrageenan has frequently been shown in studies to cause ulcers and cancer in animals. It is actually used in animal studies to *induce* ulcerative colitis because it is so effective in causing digestive distress.

Carrageenan should be avoided as much as possible, especially if you tend to have digestive problems. But carrageenan is incredibly pervasive in the modern food supply. It's in a wide variety of processed and packaged foods (like whipping cream).

It's even commonly found in seemingly "natural" foods like sour cream, cottage cheese, non-dairy milks (like almond and coconut milk), and ice cream.

Check your ingredients carefully or make these items yourself to keep carrageenan out of your diet as much as you can.

Starch. Foods that contain a lot of starch (like grains, potatoes, starchy vegetables, and unripe fruits) may or may not be irritating to your digestive system; it depends largely on your current digestive and metabolic state. For most people, starch from these foods isn't particularly irritating and can usually be eaten as part of a balanced diet.

But if you have severely compromised gut health, it can be helpful to reduce or eliminate starches for a time until you're able to heal your gut. This is because starches are made of complex carbohydrates, which may not be fully digested if you have poor gut function. The undigested portions can feed bacterial and fungal overgrowth, which will only serve to exacerbate digestive issues.

You don't necessarily have to eat a low-carb diet, however. You can get carbohydrates from fruit and honey, which provide an easily digested form of energy, as well as other protective benefits.

Note: If you have digestive problems, it may help to keep a simple log for a few weeks to see what symptoms crop up after eating certain foods. After all, you want to learn what works and what doesn't for your digestive system. This can change over time, so stay flexible.

4. EAT FOODS THAT SOOTHE AND NOURISH YOUR DIGESTIVE SYSTEM.

Avoiding irritating substances will halt the damage to your gut, but it's just as important to accelerate healing by eating foods that nourish and soothe the digestive system.

Natural sugar for energy. If you find it beneficial to reduce your starch intake, it's important to fuel your metabolism with the basic energy it needs to heal. Eating enough carbohydrates will also keep your stress hormones from climbing too high so you avoid perpetuating the cycle of stress.

You can get your carbohydrates from simple, natural sugars in fruit, fresh fruit juice, honey, and maple syrup instead. (I'll address eating these foods as part of a balanced diet, as well as common sugar myths, in upcoming chapters.)

Healing fats. The right fats are key for fighting bacterial imbalance and aiding digestion. Short- and medium-chain saturated fatty acids are easily absorbed for energy and provide protective benefits. For instance, coconut oil is primarily comprised of medium-chain fatty acids which have antibacterial, antifungal, and antiviral properties. And high quality, real butter is a natural source of butyric acid, a short-chain fatty acid that protects the integrity of the gut lining and also provides anti-inflammatory benefits. Butter is especially helpful if you can't tolerate fiber, which normally helps gut flora produce butyric acid. So if you can't (or don't) consume much fiber, butter can be tremendously healing for your digestive system.

Anti-stress proteins. Gelatin (also called collagen) is an incredibly restorative protein. Its primary amino acid, glycine, is anti-stress and anti-inflammatory. In previous centuries, cooking the whole animal was the common practice. Not only was it less wasteful, but it was also much healthier! It was part of daily life to cook broths and soups from the bones and joints, which made these foods rich in natural gelatin. Now that our diets rely more heavily on muscle meats, we've lost our primary source of gelatin protein.

You can take gelatin in powder form as a supplement. Regular gelatin needs to be mixed with a very hot liquid to dissolve, while hydrolyzed collagen can be stirred into cold or hot foods. But real, homemade broth is the best way to nourish your digestive system. It also contains important minerals and trace nutrients in addition to being a rich source of gelatin. A cup of broth with every meal can make a tremendous difference in your health.

I don't recommend most store-bought broths, as these are rarely made in a way that maximizes their gelatin and nutrient content. Plus, they are often loaded with unhealthy additives and hidden MSG (monosodium glutamate). Instead, you can make your own broth at home.

How to Make Your Own Real Broth

Bones are the key ingredient for a healthy broth. While the idea of bones, cartilage, and marrow may not get your mouth watering, it's these components that bring the amazing nutritional value to homemade broth.

Meat and vegetables can also be included in broth for flavor. Leafy greens, especially, will enhance the mineral content. You can add your favorite seasonings to the mix, like sea salt, pepper, and various spices. Don't overdo the seasoning, however, since the broth will gain its own flavor as it cooks. You can always add more later!

- To make your broth, place all of your ingredients in a large stockpot and cover with cold filtered water.
- Place the pot over medium heat until the water has reached a gentle simmer. Then adjust heat to its lowest setting and allow broth to simmer for three to four hours.
- *Remember to only allow the broth to simmer, never boil.* Boiling can botch the flavor, texture, and nutritional value of your broth.
- When your broth has finished simmering, remove it from heat and allow it to cool slightly. You'll want to strain it to separate the liquid from the solids. If you want an

exceptionally clear broth you can use a very fine strainer; but otherwise, any strainer will do.

- Strain the liquid into a large bowl or jar (preferably one with a lid or cover for easy storage). Set aside meat and vegetables to use for soups or casseroles later.

- Store the broth in the refrigerator in an airtight container overnight. The fat in the broth will harden and rise to the top of the bowl. You can skim off as much fat as you desire, but leave at least a small amount to enhance the overall flavor and texture. Of course, you can skim off all the fat and add it back in as desired later on.

- You can easily save more time by cooking large amounts of broth at once and then storing the rest in the freezer. It will keep for several months.

You can use your broth to flavor soups, sauces, gravies, and so much more. Or you can simply drink it as a metabolic supplement.

NOTE: There are some fantastic tips online for making broth in the oven, in a crockpot, and other various methods for easy broth-making. I encourage you to experiment and find a way that works best for your life.

5. DON'T EAT YOUR VEGGIES RAW

Popular mainstream advice tells us to eat more "indigestible" foods. High-fiber diets are promoted as healthy, and raw veggies are praised because they are low-calorie and "bulk" up the diet so you feel full without eating very much. Basically, we're told to fill ourselves up with non-food items so we can avoid eating *actual* food. Yeah, that sounds like it came right out of the eating disorder handbook!

The problem with raw veggies—especially salad greens and cruciferous vegetables like broccoli—is that they are packed with cellulose (an indigestible plant fiber) and anti-nutrients that can actually block the absorption of vital nutrients, contribute to poor thyroid function, and irritate the digestive system.

The human digestive system is not actually meant to break down raw vegetables. Animals that naturally consume a lot of raw greens and other vegetables are typically ruminants (having multiple stomachs to handle this difficult digestive process) like cows, goats, sheep, and camels. Other animals that eat grass and leafy greens like horses and rabbits only have one stomach, but they have a much larger cecum (a pouch at the beginning of the large intestine) than humans in order to break down cellulose.

Since humans don't have multiple stomachs or an exceptionally large cecum, it stands to reason we are simply not meant to eat a lot of leaves and grass. But the bulk of today's popular diets advocate eating a lot of salads and greens. Maybe they could use a lesson in simple human anatomy.

Broccoli and other cruciferous veggies pose another threat to your metabolism: goitrogens. Goitrogenic foods suppress thyroid function—the exact opposite of what you want for a nourished metabolism!

A Better Way to Eat Your Vegetables

But don't get the wrong idea: we're not about labeling and banning foods here. If you love raw veggies you can eat them, but I wouldn't make them the focus of your diet, especially if you have digestive issues like bloating or stomach pain after eating them. There is, however, a better way to eat vegetables so they won't stress your metabolism: just cook them!

Slow-cooked vegetables, especially when sautéed in butter and simmered in broth, are far more digestible than raw veggies. Cooking takes care of some of the concerns we discussed about raw vegetables. It neutralizes many anti-nutrients, and it also breaks down cellulose so that it's easier on the digestive system.

Cooking also partially inactivates the goitrogenic compounds in certain vegetables, but it may still be wise to avoid goitrogenic vegetables most of the time, especially if you tend to have low thyroid function.

6. KEEP IT MOVING

Constipation is not your friend. But then, you probably already knew that. Still, many people underestimate how important it is to keep your bowels moving on a regular basis.

Constipation is a stress on your digestive system, and can increase your exposure to toxins produced by pathogenic bacteria in your gut. These toxins can lead to conditions like inflammation, diabetes, and obesity—all signs of a stressed metabolism. And because the restricted blood flow and inflammation of a stressed metabolism can worsen constipation symptoms, you can quickly trigger a vicious cycle.

Addressing any metabolic cause of constipation is crucial to healing, but addressing the constipation directly can sometimes help stop the negative cycle in its tracks so you can overcome other issues. Following the advice included in this chapter (raising your metabolic rate, reducing stress, eating healthy fats, consuming broth, eating cooked vegetables, etc.) should ultimately help regulate your bowel movements. But sometimes additional steps may be needed to get things moving, especially while you're still working on healing your metabolism:

- Epsom salt baths can help relieve constipation by raising your magnesium levels. Epsom salts contain magnesium, and using them in a bath is an effective way to absorb magnesium through your skin.
- Fresh juice first thing in the morning can be especially helpful. Its magnesium and potassium are restorative and can ease constipation, but these electrolytes may

need to be balanced with a dash or two of salt. (More on the importance of salt is in Chapter 6).

- A raw carrot eaten daily is associated with improved gut function, and can help relieve constipation.

- Aged cascara sagrada bark can be used in small amounts to promote regularity. Cascara sagrada contains the compound emodin, which stimulates bowel movements. (Research has also shown that emodin has anti-inflammatory and anti-cancer properties, so cascara sagrada may prove to be beneficial beyond relieving constipation.) Only aged (not fresh) cascara sagrada bark should be used, as aging reduces potentially irritating components in the bark. Start with the smallest dose and slowly work up until you find an effective amount. You don't want to take too much and induce diarrhea, which can cause gut irritation and electrolyte imbalances.

What to Use for Indigestion

All of the above suggestions should help reduce or eliminate indigestion. But it can take time to adjust your habits and for your body to heal. In the meantime, it can help to use natural remedies for indigestion, bloating, gas, or occasional cramps after eating.

Peppermint and ginger are popular, simple, and inexpensive natural remedies for these digestive upsets. Simply have a cup of peppermint or ginger tea with meals to aid digestion and prevent any symptoms of irritation. You can also have a piece of candied ginger or natural peppermint candy after a meal for the same effect.

A Word about Probiotics

Probiotics are all the rage when it comes to improving gut health, but it's necessary to take a look at the big picture before you invest your life savings in expensive probiotic supplements.

While gut flora balance is definitely key to healing your digestive system, that doesn't necessarily mean that throwing tons of probiotics at the problem is the best way to fix it. What you really want is a metabolism that provides an environment for gut flora balance. Raising body temperature (through raising the metabolic rate), lowering inflammation, and balancing hormones are some of the factors which contribute to reduced pathogens in the gut.

Probiotic supplements also tend to focus on just a handful of known bacterial strains, whereas fermented foods (like raw sauerkraut, kimchi, or kombucha) contain a much wider spectrum of bacterial strains. There is really no need to body-slam your digestive system with large amounts of a few isolated strains of probiotics. Eating small amounts of natural, fermented foods is a more balanced way of getting probiotics into your diet.

In any case, pay close attention to how your body responds to fermented foods or probiotics, if you choose to take them. Don't just write off negative side effects (like migraines) as "die-off" symptoms. In fact, probiotic bacteria in the gut can produce high levels of lactic acid, which is linked to migraines. This may be a sign that your digestive system can't properly cope with the presence of additional bacteria. So, as always, listen to your body!

Chapter 5:
A Balanced Plan
for Eating

BY NOW, I HOPE I'VE CONVINCED YOU to leave dieting behind and approach your eating habits in a new way. But in order to give up old habits, you have to replace them with new ones. And for a nourished metabolism, it's not as hard as you might think. What you really need is *balance*. I know this is practically a foreign word in today's society, but avoiding extremes is going to be one of the most effective ways to boost your metabolic health and stop the damage caused by high stress hormones.

In ideal conditions, your body should have access to plenty of energy (calories), all three macronutrients (carbohydrates, fat, and protein), and micronutrients (vitamins and minerals) in relatively balanced amounts. Sure, your body is technically capable of making its own fuel if it's required, but this is a sort of emergency back-up plan for when the right balance isn't coming from your diet. It's not something you should be forcing your body to do every day.

If you want to stress out your metabolism, start denying it some of the most basic elements it needs to survive. This simple act of deprivation is enough to trigger the release of stress hormones and all the accompanying side effects. Why? Because the body uses the stress hormones adrenaline and cortisol to access alternate sources of energy (i.e. get glucose from protein or ketones from fat).

In the beginning, these deprivation diets can produce weight loss and even some positive side effects that make it appear as if they're helping. But that's just the initial surge of adrenaline and cortisol talking.

If you've been on any of these diets, you know that after a few weeks, some of the fun feelings start to wear off. You might be in a bad mood more often, or you might notice feeling cold and not sleeping well. And of course, weight loss begins to stall as your metabolism downregulates to handle the stress.

That's the good ole False Feel-Good Phase wearing off. And

this is your body telling you to stop all this deprivation and start a more balanced approach to eating instead.

STOP THE RESTRICT AND REPENT CYCLE

The modern diet mentality is one of the biggest hurdles to overcome if you want to eat for a nourished metabolism. We have become convinced as a culture that we must blame food (or certain foods) for our problems, which means the only solution is to restrict and avoid as much as we can. Vegans blame animal foods, low-carbers blame bread, and low-fat folks blame butter. Different groups have different scapegoats, but the method is the same: restrict, restrict, restrict.

It's not uncommon for people to get so wrapped up in what they *shouldn't* eat that thinking about food completely takes over their lives. Their every waking moment is consumed by planning, preparing, worrying, and obsessing over food.

The problem is that restrictive diets almost always backfire. They consume our thoughts and our energy to point of becoming a major source of stress in our lives. And often the way we relieve this unbearable stress is by throwing our restrictions out the window and binging on the very foods we've been restricting.

This is what I call the **Restrict and Repent Cycle**. You restrict a type of food (or food in general) so stringently that you eventually give up and eat everything you've been denying yourself. But this only leads to a feeling of failure. So you repent and shame yourself, and vow to restrict your diet even more ruthlessly tomorrow. You could go into deep psychological analysis on why this pattern seems to be so inevitable (there are many articles and books on the subject), but I think it's important to focus on *why this pattern needs to end.*

The Restrict and Repent Cycle is a source of great stress on our bodies and minds. In fact, for some of us, **it is the single most damaging source of stress in our lives.** Replacing this kind of negative mental pattern is crucial for reducing your overall stress load and overcoming food issues.

Not only is this cycle stressful, it also denies you the right to listen to your body. A restrictive diet tells you to follow a rigid plan without the freedom to adjust as your individual body responds to what you feed it. Sometimes those late-night binges are just the inevitable outcome of not listening to your body! Then you tend to overcompensate and eat too much of what you're craving, when overeating isn't really what your body wanted. This leads to feelings of guilt and repentance, where you once again convince yourself that you can't listen to your body (because it's obviously crazy!).

Over time this, cycle completely impairs your ability to listen to what your body is telling you. Pretty soon you can't tell if you're hungry or if you're full, if you need more fruit or more fat. You constantly pin your body in a struggle against a plan. Sometimes the plan wins... sometimes your body wins. But in the end, you get the feeling that your body is an enemy you're fighting with, instead of an incredible biological system with its own built-in wisdom.

So instead of restricting and repenting, I like to encourage a more positive and balanced pattern that encourages you to listen to your body. I call it the **Replace and Rebuild Principle**.

BALANCED EATING PRINCIPLE #1: REPLACE AND REBUILD

Most eating plans place an inordinate amount of focus on what you *shouldn't* eat. The focus is always on restricting and limiting. Not only is this negative approach an immediate downer, its very premise triggers the Restrict and Repent Cycle.

That's why I recommend that you limit dietary restrictions as much as possible. If there are some habits you can improve or better choices you can make, then that's something you can work toward. But you do not need to ban foods, limit your food choices, or set a ton of rigid boundaries about what you can and cannot eat.

Instead, think in terms of replacing. And what are good replacement foods? **Foods that rebuild your body.** This is the foundation of the *Replace and Rebuild Principle*.

Healthy food is food that helps your body rebuild. You want to rebuild your energy levels, hormone levels, lean body mass structure, and your nutrient levels. The right foods supply your body with what it needs to keep all of these at their best.

BALANCED EATING PRINCIPLE #2: LISTEN TO YOUR BODY

There are hundreds of diet books on the market. And they all tell you what to eat, when to eat it and how to eat it. They say the most important thing is to follow their eating rules. I respectfully disagree.

The most important thing is to *listen to your body*. This means:

- Eat what you love.
- Love what you eat.
- Pay attention to how your body responds.
- Adjust your diet as needed to get the best response from your body.

Some people are afraid to listen to their bodies because they've been told by some diet guru that their body can't be trusted. They've been told their body wants to eat an entire chocolate cake and lay around on the couch all day not moving.

I say go ahead! Eat a ton of chocolate cake and lay around on the couch all day. Feel better? Yeah, I didn't think so. Your body is telling you that wasn't such a good idea, right? That's called biofeedback, and Chapter 10 of this book is dedicated to helping you learn to listen to it.

BALANCED EATING PRINCIPLE #3: ENERGY VERSUS NUTRIENTS

Your body needs a careful balance of energy versus nutrients. Too much energy without enough nutrients, and you wind up with problems connected to nutrient deficiencies. Plenty of nutrients without enough energy leads to a slow metabolism and its associated side effects.

The key is to get the right amount of both. Eat enough food to fuel your metabolic rate and your daily activities, and make sure those foods are supplying your body with the nutrients it needs to function optimally.

This doesn't mean that every bite you eat must be nutrient-dense. There is still a lot of room for flexibility. You just want to make sure the bulk of your diet is supplying you with a balance of energy-rich and nutrient-rich foods. For instance, white rice is a relatively neutral food. It's a great source of easily digested energy, but it also contains virtually no vitamins and minerals. If you eat it as a side to a hearty stew made with grass-fed beef and real broth, suddenly you've got a meal that supplies you with energy *and* nutrients.

That's just one basic example, but the underlying principle is important: **Eat a variety of foods that balance energy with**

nutrients, and your metabolic health will be supported by everything it needs.

BALANCED EATING PRINCIPLE #4: EAT A BALANCE OF CARBS, FAT, AND PROTEIN

Low-fat. Low-carb. High-fat. High-protein. Take your pick. People like to argue about macronutrients. It seems to be one of the favorite hobbies of the health-conscious. How much fat? How many carbs? How much protein?

Plenty of people like to pretend there's a "magic" macronutrient composition that is right for everyone; but in my experience, oversimplification leads only to frustration and could even result in stressing your metabolism. If you want an eating plan for life, forget fad diets that restrict macronutrients. Instead, eat balanced!

The basic structure you want in a diet is a balance of carbohydrates, proteins, and fats. You want some of each every day, preferably some of each at every meal and snack. These macronutrients are complementary, aiding in the optimal absorption and utilization of each other to promote a nourished metabolism.

I believe your body can help you find that sweet spot of the right amount of carbs, fat, and protein for *you*. Having said that, many people have asked me for a guide so they can get an idea of what they should be moving toward. We like to see things in numbers. It helps give us a target to shoot for so we feel like we're meeting our nutritional goals. So here is a rough guide that you can use as a starting place. I absolutely encourage you to listen to your body and tweak it as much as needed.

CARBOHYDRATES: Eat a *minimum* of 1 to 1.5 grams per pound of body weight.

> *Example: If you weigh 150 lbs, eat **at least** 150 - 225 carbohydrates per day. (If you are physically active, you may need more than this.)*

PROTEIN: Eat a *minimum* of 0.5 grams per pound of body weight.

> *Example: If you weigh 150 lbs, eat **at least** 75 grams of protein per day. (Again, if you are active, you may need more.)*

FAT: Dietary fat is a heated topic, but the type of fat you eat is more important than the exact number of grams. (We'll discuss healthy fats later in this chapter.) The body needs fat to utilize important fat-soluble vitamins, produce hormones, enhance immunity, and much more.

Listen to your body to determine the right amount of fat in your diet. Too little and you'll tend to feel unsatisfied or empty after a meal. Too much and you may experience indigestion, bloating, and stomach pains. Some people do better with more fat in their diets, while others do better with less; and most of us fall somewhere in the middle.

TOTAL DAILY CALORIE INTAKE: Most women need at least 2,000 calories per day to support their metabolic health and activity, while men typically need no less than 2,500 calories per day. These numbers will vary based on your metabolism, size (height and weight), and activity levels. More importantly, **eat when your body is hungry, and eat the amount that makes you feel satisfied and comfortably full.**

IMPORTANT! All of these numbers are only meant as a rough guide. Be flexible and make adjustments based on your biofeedback. Figure out the mix that works for *your* body and *your* lifestyle. The only magic number is the one that works for *you.*

"BUT AREN'T CARBOHYDRATES BAD FOR YOU?!?"

The myth that carbohydrates are unhealthy and fattening is one of the biggest dietary misconceptions in our culture today. The theory is that high blood sugar is bad, therefore carbohydrates are bad because they can raise your blood sugar. While it makes sense on the surface, this theory ignores a few very important biological facts:

- Cells in your body rely on a constant and steady supply of energy from glucose (blood sugar) to function optimally. While you don't want your blood sugar chronically high, you don't want it too low either. Carbohydrates fuel activity within your cells, which in turn fuels metabolic function.
- The glycemic index isn't everything. Carbohydrates eaten

with a balance of protein and fat enter the bloodstream more slowly and give your metabolism a steady supply of its favorite energy source: glucose. Most glycemic index models only look at how specific foods affect your blood sugar when eaten *alone*. When you eat balanced meals, the whole game changes.

- Stress hormones like cortisol and epinephrine can actually raise your blood sugar (it's part of the fight-or-flight response) by breaking down proteins in your body (i.e. bone and muscle mass) and turning them into glucose. Low blood sugar can actually raise your stress hormone levels to facilitate this process.

- Eating carbohydrates can lower stress hormones by raising insulin and, therefore, actually help blood sugar reach normal levels, while simultaneously reducing other negative side effects of high stress hormones. Insulin gets a bad rap, but it's insulin imbalance that is the problem. You don't want your insulin levels too high *or* too low. Your body needs normal insulin levels to function properly.

- Research has demonstrated that low-carb diets lower thyroid hormone levels, T3 levels specifically. Thyroid health is the center of metabolic health; and downregulating thyroid hormones will, in turn, downregulate the metabolism. In short, low-carb diets lower your metabolic rate.

Figuring out the right balance of carbohydrates in your diet is crucial for improving your metabolic health. If your metabolism is stressed, it may help to divide your carbohydrates into small, balanced meals throughout the day to promote blood-sugar balance.

As your metabolism heals and stress-hormone levels normalize, you may find you can eat more carbohydrates in one sitting and still maintain balanced blood sugar levels. But cutting out carbohydrates to balance your blood sugar can actually have the opposite effect over time, as your body increases stress-hormone production to make up for the lack of glucose in your diet. Basically, chronically high stress hormones can lead to chronically high blood-sugar levels, the unintended side effect of the low-carb diet.

WHY WHOLE GRAINS MAY NOT BE YOUR FRIEND

Whole grains are better for you, right? Wrong! Or at least, not necessarily. Eating whole grains may not be the best way to nourish your metabolism, and here's why:

- The bran and germ can present problems. As we discussed in the previous chapter, fiber can cause digestive issues in many individuals. In whole grains, the bran and germ provide fiber that can potentially irritate your digestive tract and cause inflammation. They are best avoided if you have poor gut health.

- The bran and germ of whole grains also contain polyunsaturated fats, which makes them vulnerable to oxidation and rancidity.
- Nutrients come with anti-nutrients. The reason whole grains are considered "healthy" is because they contain some vitamins and minerals. But what whole-grain enthusiasts usually don't tell you is that these nutrients are accompanied by anti-nutrients such as phytic acid.
- Phytic acid binds to minerals and prevents your body from absorbing them, which negates some of the nutrient content in whole grains and may even prevent the absorption of nutrients from the other foods you're eating. Soaking and sprouting may help to reduce the anti-nutrients in whole grains, although this process may not be practical for everyone.

So, does this mean you can *never* eat whole grains? Of course not! It just means it can be helpful to consider the pros and cons before you decide how much to include them in your diet. And if you do use whole grains regularly, you might want to look into using traditional preparation methods like soaking, fermenting, and sprouting.

THE RIGHT CARBS FOR YOUR BODY

The right carbs are the carbs that work for *you*. I know, that's not as easy as me just telling you exactly what to eat. But the thing is, only you live in *your* body; and only you can decide which carbohydrates work for your body and your life.

But to help you on your journey of figuring out which carbs work for you, here is a quick rundown of the pros and cons of a few top carbohydrate sources:

FRUIT. Easily digested, not likely to irritate your digestive system, especially if cooked or juiced. Contains a good balance of carbohydrates with vitamins and minerals, especially vitamin C, folate, magnesium, and potassium, as well as other protective nutrients like flavonoids. Fresh-pressed juice can be particularly helpful for condensed energy and nutrition. Fruit is a great, nutrient-dense way to get your carbs. Eating too much peel or too many seeds may be irritating to your digestive system, so avoid overdoing these.

POTATOES. One of the friendlier starches, potatoes are a good source of quality protein, as well as many vitamins and minerals. They are also gluten free and tend to be more easily digested than grains. Consider potatoes a top-notch starch. (There are anti-nutrients in the peel that may be a problem if you eat a *lot* of potatoes. If you're concerned, just peel them.) Other root vegetables and tubers should be considered similar to potatoes.

WHITE RICE. I recommend white rice, since even soaked brown rice tends to have high phytic acid levels. White rice is a relatively benign carbohydrate. Although it contains few nutrients and should be paired with more nutrient-dense foods, it is also less irritating than other grains, especially glutenous grains.

CORN. Also gluten free, corn can be one of the more easily-digested grains, depending on how it's processed. Corn boiled or soaked in an alkaline solution (the traditional preparation method) tends to improve the availability of its nutrients and make it more digestible.

HONEY, MAPLE SYRUP, CANE SUGAR, ETC. Sweeteners provide energy just like other carbohydrates. The advantage of sweeteners is they are easily broken down because they contain mostly short-chain carbohydrates like glucose and fructose. This can be useful to those with digestive issues, who need energy but have a hard time handling complex carbohydrates. Some unrefined sugar sources like raw honey, real maple syrup, and date sugar also contain trace nutrients. (Sugars of all kinds have been demonized in the health world, so I'll be addressing some of the myths about sugar in the next chapter.)

WHEAT AND OTHER GLUTENOUS GRAINS. Gluten is one of the latest scapegoats in popular diet books, but I don't recommend banning all gluten from your diet unless you are certain of an allergy or severe intolerance. There's nothing wrong with enjoying some wheat products as part of a varied, nutritious diet. Whole wheat and other similar grains may benefit from a soak in an acidic solution overnight before being cooked, or you can choose to eat refined grains to avoid the bran and germ altogether—just eat plenty of nutrient-dense foods as well. Slow-rise breads and well-cooked oats fall into the category of decent grains to eat in moderation. The extent you include these foods in your diet should be based on your own biofeedback. Some people find they can eat small amounts daily; others can enjoy them a couple times a week without any problem. It's up to you to determine what works for your body.

BEANS AND LEGUMES. Beans do contain some important nutrients like B vitamins; but they present a few problems as well, especially when eaten in large quantities. Beans have a high fiber and anti-nutrient content, as well as estrogenic compounds that may exacerbate hormonal imbalances. Beans should *always* be soaked overnight and cooked very well before eating. Definitely listen to your body with these. Some experience a lot of digestive complaints that are solved just by reducing or eliminating beans from their diet. Do what works for you!

Remember, it's not about excluding or restricting any of these foods from your diet, but eating a variety of real food and adjusting as needed according to your body's response.

THE RIGHT FATS FOR A NOURISHED METABOLISM

Next to bashing carbohydrates, diet gurus also like to bash saturated fats. This is fueled by a cultural misconception that saturated fats are bad, while polyunsaturated vegetable oils are healthy fats.

But this is ultimately a myth–one that definitely stresses your metabolism. Eating the *right* fats is an important key to nourishing your metabolism, but the right fats may not be what you think. In fact, what mainstream ideology calls the "right" fats are actually the wrong ones! I'm talking about "healthy" polyunsaturated oils. In reality, vegetable oils are doing you more harm than good; and here's why:

- The main difference between polyunsaturated fats and other fats (like monounsaturated and saturated fats) is their structure.

- For example, monounsaturated fatty acids are linked by one double bond, but polyunsaturated fatty acids are linked by multiple double bonds.

- This multiple-bond structure is very unstable and oxidizes easily. This wreaks havoc on the cells in your body. It contributes to oxidative stress, which is linked to heart disease, cancer, Alzheimer's disease, diabetes and premature aging (just to name a few).

The instability of polyunsaturated fats is especially volatile during any kind of processing. Even small amounts of light, moisture, air, or heat damage polyunsaturated fatty acids. These oils can't withstand exposure to heat when used for cooking, and yet they are the most popular choice for cooking in most restaurants and in packaged foods. Vegetable oils are also typically bleached and deodorized with chemicals to cover up the fact that the oils went rancid during processing.

Rancid fats wreak havoc in your body through oxidative stress, which harms your health at a metabolic level. These unstable fats have an anti-thyroid effect on the body, meaning they downregulate the metabolism. These anti-metabolic effects are demonstrated in studies that show polyunsaturated fats can promote diabetes and weight gain.

Unfortunately, the vegetable-oil producers have spent a lot of money marketing and lobbying to promote a positive image of their oils, which explains why the idea of "healthy vegetable oils" is so commonly accepted. But this message flies in the face of historical and scientific evidence which shows vegetable oils should *not* make up a significant part of our diets.

AVOID HYDROGENATED OIL, SHORTENING, AND MARGARINE

Hydrogenation turns liquid oil into solid oil. But just because margarine looks like real butter doesn't make it real food! Hydrogenated oil is full of trans-fatty acids, which research has linked to degenerative conditions like:

- Heart disease
- Colon cancer
- Breast cancer
- Stroke

Lesson of the day? Just skip the hydrogenated oils.

STICK WITH TRADITIONAL FATS

Before industrial vegetable oils became the norm, fats traditionally used by our ancestors included butter, ghee, cream, beef tallow, lard, and tropical oils like coconut oil. What do these fats have in common? They all contain a lot of saturated fat!

Traditional cultures did not liberally use vegetable oils in their diets. Keep in mind that these cultures often exhibited excellent health and were not plagued by modern degenerative diseases. Weston A. Price noted in his book *Nutrition and Physical Degeneration* that industrial vegetable oils were one of the modern foods that brought health problems to traditional people when they started using them in their diets. We should take a hint from our ancestors and ditch the industrial fats.

Surprisingly, heart disease and other degenerative conditions have only become more common since vegetable oils have replaced traditional fats in our diets. I think our ancestors were onto something, don't you?

FOR THE LOVE OF BUTTER

Butter is one of my favorite fats. Not only is it incredibly delicious, it also provides some pretty great health benefits—especially if it's grass-fed butter from pastured cows. Butter is rich in fat-soluble vitamins like vitamin A and vitamin K2 in a highly bioavailable state that our bodies can easily utilize. These vitamins work together with other fat-soluble vitamins (like vitamin D and vitamin E) to promote immunity, thyroid health, bone health, and much more. Butter also contains protective fatty acids like butyric acid, which can be a vital nutrient for improving your gut health.

COCONUT OIL: THE SUPER FAT

Next to butter, coconut oil is the fat source I recommend the most. Coconut oil is comprised almost entirely of medium-chain saturated fatty acids that provide astounding metabolic benefits.

The fatty acids in coconut oil are very stable and resistant to oxidation, which makes them perfect for counteracting the oxidative effects of polyunsaturated oils. These fatty acids have been shown to promote heart health and a healthy body weight.

The unique structure of coconut oil's fatty acids allow them to be converted easily by the liver into energy, which makes coconut oil the perfect food for those who need an easily digested form of energy (as is often the case in those with low metabolic function). This efficient energy conversion paired with its antioxidant properties may explain why coconut oil is so well-known for nourishing thyroid and metabolic health.

PRESENTING LAURIC ACID (BROUGHT TO YOU BY COCONUT OIL)

Lauric acid is an important medium-chain fatty acid found mainly in coconut oil. Pure coconut oil contains about 50% lauric acid, which makes it the most abundant natural source of lauric acid on earth.

When lauric acid is present in the body, it's converted into monolaurin, a compound which has potent antiviral, antimicrobial, antiprotozoal, and antifungal properties. It acts by disrupting the lipid membranes in organisms like fungi, bacteria, and viruses, thus destroying them. Specifically, the compound monolaurin is an effective treatment for candida albicans and fungal infections like ringworm and athlete's foot. Monolaurin also targets bacterial infections, as well as lipid-coated viruses like herpes, the measles, influenza, and hepatitis C.

Plus, lauric acid is essentially non-toxic, which gives it a distinct advantage over modern pharmaceutical drugs that are typically used to fight viruses, bacterial infections, and fungal infections. (I'd rather down some coconut oil than conventional drugs if I had the choice!)

Without a plentiful source of lauric acid, the body cannot produce monolaurin, and all of these important benefits are lost.

And *that* is why I'm a big fan of coconut oil.

Here are some changes you can make to eat more of the right fats for a nourished metabolism:

1. **AVOID VEGETABLE OILS.** Don't use soy, corn, cottonseed, or canola oils if you can avoid them. Good quality olive oil is fine in moderation. (It has some polyunsaturated fats, but not a lot).

2. **EAT REAL BUTTER.** Margarine and other spreads are made with vegetable oil (sometimes the hydrogenated kind—yuck!). Stick with butter without additives and from pastured cows, if possible.

3. **CHANGE YOUR COOKING OIL.** Polyunsaturated fats are simply too unstable to heat. Switch to butter, coconut oil, ghee, and other stable saturated fats. Using olive oil for cooking on occasion is safe, too, but it's not as stable as the above fats.

4. **AVOID PROCESSED FOODS.** Unhealthy vegetable oils and trans fats are further incentive to avoid packaged food products. Stick with the real thing, and you'll have more control over which fats you consume.

5. **On the same note, AVOID COMMERCIAL SALAD DRESSINGS, MAYONNAISE, AND OTHER FATTY CONDIMENTS.** Unless otherwise noted, these are generally made with refined vegetable oils.

6. **GO EASY ON THE NUTS**. While nuts may be hailed as a health food by many experts, when eaten in excess, nuts can easily push your polyunsaturated fat intake over the limit. A few servings a week is more than enough. Hazelnuts and macadamia nuts are the most forgiving since these contain the lowest polyunsaturated fat content.

Q. WHAT IF EATING FAT MAKES ME FEEL SICK?

A. This is not uncommon if you've been eating a low-fat diet. When our bodies have been deprived of fat for a long time, the art of digesting fats is forgotten! You can help pump up your digestive juices by taking one to two teaspoons of apple cider vinegar before meals, taking digestive bitters after a meal, or eating lacto-fermented foods like sauerkraut with your meal. If you're not used to eating much fat, increase your intake of easily digested fats like butter and coconut oil slowly over a period of weeks. This will allow your body to adjust.

Remember to allow your body to dictate what amount of fat works for you in your daily diet. If you're eating a lot of fat, and you feel bloated or sick to your stomach after a meal, you might just be eating more fat than your body wants!

THE RIGHT BALANCE OF PROTEIN

Protein is made of amino acids, the building blocks that make up our muscles; our bones; our organs; and even the brain chemicals that make us feel happy, emotionally stable, and energetic.

Adequate protein intake is essential for keeping stress hormones low. If your diet doesn't supply enough amino acids to maintain the function of its vital systems, the body will release cortisol to mobilize amino acids from your lean tissues. This is a great survival mechanism if you're in a famine; but in everyday life, it leads to chronically high stress-hormone levels and suppressed metabolic function. Plus, it's eating away at your lean mass, which is definitely not good!

While it's crucial to get enough protein to support your metabolic function, the quality of protein you eat is important, too.

FOODS FOR A BALANCED PROTEIN INTAKE

DAIRY (MILK, CHEESE, YOGURT, ETC.). Dairy is high in protein as well as vitamin A, vitamin K2, B vitamins, calcium, and other important nutrients. Try to avoid dairy products from cows given pesticide-heavy diets, antibiotics, and hormones. Dairy from pastured (grass-fed) cows is preferable because it is far more nutritious. You can also try raw (unpasteurized, unhomogenized) dairy, which is often better tolerated because its enzymes and nutrients are unprocessed and intact. Goat milk may be well tolerated if cow milk is not.

EGGS. Eggs (especially from free-range hens) definitely fit the bill for a nutritious source of protein. They are loaded with nutrients like B vitamins, vitamin A, vitamin D, selenium, zinc, and choline. The catch? The nutrition is all in the yolk! So make sure to eat *whole* eggs. (Don't worry, research has shown that eating whole eggs does not negatively affect your cholesterol levels.)

HIGH QUALITY MEATS. Meats raised with traditional methods have a better nutritional profile and a lower polyunsaturated fat content. Grass-fed beef is an especially good source of B vitamins and zinc. Meat is high in protein, but meat consumption should be balanced with broth or gelatin (see below).

REAL BONE BROTH. Old-fashioned broths and stocks made from gelatin-rich bones and joints of meat animals (typically beef or chicken) are very nutritious and filled with an easily digested form of protein–especially helpful if you have trouble with digestion.

SEAFOOD. A good source of minerals and trace nutrients, seafood is also high in protein. Shrimp and oysters contain high levels of nutrients like zinc, copper, and B vitamins. There are concerns about toxic heavy metals in seafood, which is something to consider and probably makes it best to consume seafood in moderation.

NUTS AND LEGUMES. Beans and nuts are sometimes a favorite source of protein for vegetarians, but they do present a few concerns due to their high-fiber, anti-nutrient, and polyunsaturated-fat content. They are fine in moderation, but should not be a primary source of protein.

GRAINS AND STARCHES. These contain some protein that can help augment your primary protein intake, but I wouldn't recommend relying on them as your main source of protein simply because it's not as practical or nutritious as other sources of protein.

PROTEIN POWDERS. I do not recommend most commercially produced protein powders. They are typically highly processed and refined, contain few nutrients outside of protein, and do not provide the right balance of amino acids. The only protein supplement I recommend is high-quality gelatin or hydrolyzed collagen.

THE BENEFITS OF GLYCINE (IT'S WHAT MAKES GELATIN SO GREAT!)

Different amino acids serve different functions in the body, but the modern diet neglects one of the most important anti-stress amino acids: glycine.

What is the primary amino acid in gelatin? You guessed it: glycine! Here's why I consider glycine the ultimate anti-stress amino acid:

- Glycine has been shown to have remarkable anti-inflammatory benefits, which are especially helpful to anyone under stress or with impaired digestion.

- It has also been shown to improve conditions related to seizures.
- Glycine has been used with success to improve the symptoms of schizophrenia, which may be a statement to its importance for mental health.
- Research indicates that glycine can protect against liver damage and offer anti-cancer benefits.
- Glycine can help balance blood sugar levels by working with insulin to help the body use glucose properly (which improves energy conversion–i.e. metabolic function!).

This wide range of benefits points to glycine nourishing the metabolism on a basic level. This fits perfectly with the traditional practices of preparing animal protein to include glycine-rich gelatin. And it makes sense that we should do the same.

One way to consume more gelatin is to eat real broth more often, especially when you eat meats, in order to balance out your protein intake.

You can also supplement your protein intake with powdered gelatin to increase your glycine intake. High quality powdered gelatin or hydrolyzed collagen is an excellent source of glycine and a good way to consume a balance of proteins, especially if you don't tend to consume much broth.

I personally get about 30–50 grams of protein from gelatin every day, which makes up about half of my overall protein intake.

FOR PETE'S SAKE, STOP THE SOY!

Although warnings about the safety of soy consumption are becoming more mainstream, soy is still considered a health food by many. Even the medical community—who should be aware of the side effects of soy consumption—still recommends this food as a great vegetarian source of protein and nutrients. But I beg to differ.

I like to call soy an "anti-food." That may sound harsh to you, but soy can have a profoundly negative impact on our metabolic health. Here are just some of the properties that I believe make soy an anti-food:

PHYTOESTROGENS. These are essentially plant hormones. I know a lot of people who buy organic soy milk to avoid hormones, not realizing that soy provides its own plant hormones! Phytoestrogens interfere with normal hormone regulation and can lead to imbalances tied to infertility, low sex drive, reproductive cancers, and more.

GOITROGENS. Soy is high in goitrogens, or thyroid-suppressing substances; and the particular goitrogens in soy are not neutralized with cooking. This makes soy products anti-thyroid, and therefore anti-metabolic.

TRYPSIN INHIBITORS. The enzyme trypsin is important for protein assimilation, so these inhibitors interfere with protein absorption—ironic, considering soy is supposed to be a valuable protein source. These trypsin inhibitors have led to pancreatic disorders (including cancer) in test animals.

PHYTIC ACID. Soy contains very high levels of phytic acid, which interferes with the use of valuable nutrients. Traditionally, soy was only eaten in highly fermented forms, which reduces the effects of phytic acid in soy.

Soy consumption should typically be limited, especially for anyone susceptible to poor thyroid function and hormonal imbalances. Processed soy foods are a particular concern because they're often loaded with chemicals and additives to make them taste and feel like "normal" food. Soy consumption should be minimal, fermented when possible; and avoid the processed stuff altogether.

ORGANIC FOOD: SORTING THROUGH FACT AND FICTION

The organic food movement has been gaining momentum for decades. A few years ago, sourcing organic ingredients was next to impossible in my local market. Now, there are organic foods showing up left and right, with more coming each day. It's exciting to see the organic lifestyle gaining popularity, but at the same time it's all too easy to get caught up in the movement and assume that organic equals healthy.

The most beneficial aspect of organic food is what it does *not* contain: a boatload of chemical pesticides, fertilizers, antibiotics, and added hormones. Conventional diets contain far more of these chemicals than our bodies are meant to handle. And forcing our bodies to try and contend with all the side effects of being exposed to these toxins is a new and profound source of stress.

For instance, hundreds of pesticides have been tested and confirmed to contain estrogenic or anti-androgenic properties. These components can disrupt natural hormone levels and cause imbalances, which can lead to metabolic stress.

WHAT ORGANIC MEANS

- Organic produce, meat, and dairy must be grown or raised without chemical pesticides, fertilizers, antibiotics, or hormones, and cannot be genetically modified (GMO).
- Ingredients in organic packaged foods have to be at least 95% organic by weight.

WHAT ORGANIC DOES NOT MEAN

- Organic produce, meat, and dairy may or may not be grown or raised using humane methods that maximize nutrition (i.e. grass-fed beef).
- Ingredients in organic packaged foods may or may not be healthy (they can still contain a lot of "empty" calories), and additives like carrageenan may still be present.

The point is that while buying organic food has definite

advantages, it is not the only factor in determining what constitutes healthy food. Knowing *where* your food comes from and *how* it was grown or raised is also important. Sometimes the easiest way to do this is to go down to your local farmer's markets and get familiar with farmers in your area who practice methods that promote more nutritious foods while also avoiding the use of toxic chemicals, antibiotics, and added hormones.

"WHAT IF I CAN'T AFFORD ORGANIC?"

Don't stress about it! Seriously, the foundation of nourishing your metabolism means avoiding stress whenever possible. If it's not affordable or practical for you to source organic or local foods, then *don't worry about what you can't do.* Find a way to do the best you can, and realize that there will always be limits to what we are able to accomplish at any given time.

There have been several periods in the last few years that my time or my budget was constrained to the point that it was no longer feasible for me to buy organic and local foods. At times like these, just do the best you can with what you have by prioritizing nutritious foods and avoiding the worst offenders like heavily processed foods, vegetable oils, and hydrogenated fats.

But being on a budget doesn't necessarily mean you have to sacrifice the quality of your diet. There are some incredible resources online that talk about some truly creative and ingenious ways to work healthy foods into even the most meager budget.

In the end, be flexible and forgiving with your food choices. Life comes in waves and ebbs; there are times when eating well will be easy and other times... not so much. Whatever you do, don't let the obsession of eating the "perfect" diet become a source of stress and anxiety in your life!

Chapter 6:
Salt, Sugar, and
Water Myths

Salt, sugar, and water are three of the most misunderstood substances on the planet. They have been labeled and mislabeled about as many times as you could imagine, yet old myths seem to hang on into the new century. It's time to take a step back and consider what each does for us metabolically before we make any blanket judgments.

SALT MYTHS

Every cell in the body requires salt; and countless functions depend on the presence of sodium, including everything from blood sugar regulation to bone density to circulatory health. And because we lose salt constantly during the day through urine and perspiration, it's important that we replenish it.

Cravings for salty food are almost universally common in our culture, but it's still politically incorrect to salt your food to taste. Restrictive low-sodium diets are another darling of the diet industry, probably because they result in quick water loss which may fool dieters into thinking their fad diet is working. In reality, it could be endangering their health.

LOW-SALT DIETS CAN PUT YOUR HEALTH AT RISK

Sodium is often viewed as one of the deadly ingredients in our food. But contrary to popular belief, normal sodium consumption is not linked to a higher death rate. In fact, several studies point to a higher death rate in those who eat *less* salt. Let me say it again: **a low-salt diet is tied to a higher mortality rate**. And those who eat *more* salt tend to live longer and experience a lower rate of heart attack and stroke.

For example, a study in 2011 looked at sodium intake in 30,000 individuals and found those who consumed between 4,000 and 6,000 milligrams of sodium per day—more than double the current recommendations—were at the least risk for heart disease and stroke. Those who consumed a very high *or* very low amount of sodium were at a higher risk. Moderation seems to be key.

Another indicator of the metabolic benefit of sodium is its ability to help the body process blood sugar. Insulin resistance (an inability to process blood sugar) actually increases on a low-salt diet.

Essentially, a low-salt diet throws your metabolic systems out of whack and puts you at risk for the very conditions these diets are meant to correct. Why? Because salt plays a very important role in metabolic balance.

How Salt Nourishes Your Metabolism

Salt acts as a thermogenic substance in the body, which means it increases your energy expenditure and heat production. In short, **salt actually raises your metabolic rate**.

This is why eating enough salt is an important key to achieving a nourished metabolism: by lowering stress hormones and raising the metabolic rate, salt can resolve a myriad of metabolic issues like cold hands and feet, low moods, poor stress tolerance, insomnia, and many more. It also works to lower stress hormones and also raises oxytocin levels, which can lift your moods and give you a feeling of well-being.

What Type of Salt is Best?

Table salt is typically full of additives and anti-caking agents. Many versions of commercial salt also contain aluminum derivatives, which are known to be highly toxic.

Sourcing higher quality salt doesn't have to be complicated. Regular canning salt, for instance, is an inexpensive alternative to table salt. It contains no additives and is basically pure sodium. Provided the rest of your diet supplies you with a good variety of minerals, canning salt can be a simple and affordable way to salt your food.

You can also try some of the various sea salts and natural rock salts on the market. They are generally much more expensive, but some contain a more balanced mineral profile. Keep in mind that the source of your salt makes a difference. Some of these salts may be too high in iron and other metals which are not desirable.

HOW MUCH SALT DO WE NEED?

Once you have a good quality salt, there is only one basic rule for how much salt you should consume: salt your food to taste.

Someone with a stressed metabolism will naturally enjoy more salt on their food, whereas someone with a nourished metabolism may prefer less. And because your metabolic needs can vary from day to day, it's important to let your individual body clue you in on how much sodium it needs.

It's important to allow your body to dictate how much salt you use in your diet. Most people with a stressed metabolism naturally gravitate toward saltier foods, and won't mind the taste of a salt-water mixture or even putting a little salt straight on their tongues.

If this is the case, you may benefit from taking an additional ⅛ to ¼ teaspoon of salt with a glass of water once in the morning, once in the evening, and throughout the day as needed. I do this on a regular basis, and I can really feel the difference! The salt can be mixed right into the water or you can take it like I do: straight on the tongue and then chased with some water or other beverage.

If you are working on nourishing your metabolism, as time passes, you may notice that the salty taste is less appealing, or you may start desiring more water-rich foods like fruit instead of salty foods. This is just a natural cue from your body about your sodium needs.

Salt with Wisdom

As beneficial as salt is, more (and more and more) is not always better. Although the body can be forgiving with salt intake, excess is not beneficial and has its own risks. That is why it's so important to listen to your body and let it dictate your salt intake. (Don't force-feed yourself salt all day, every day!)

Please note: For most people with a stressed metabolism, eating salt is highly beneficial and has few side effects. But there are a few exceptions: those with heart disease, hypertension, or kidney disease should consult with a professional first, as salt may be contraindicated. As always, closely monitor how your body reacts to any substance or food, and work with a medical professional if you have any concerns.

THE Nourished METABOLISM

SUGAR MYTHS

I think a little rational logic is needed on the topic of sugar. But that's not easy when all you hear from diet books, talk show hosts, and even your Aunt Linda is that sugar is horrible, evil, addictive, and fattening. Almost every single health guru agrees on at least one thing: sugar is the bane of modern society. It's been called a poison and even a drug. Some folks want to tax it. Some even want to outlaw it.

The problem? It's your body's favorite fuel.

In fact, your body will find a way to get sugar to your cells even if you don't eat it. It will break down complex carbohydrates into simple sugars. And if you don't eat carbohydrates, your body will turn to proteins (from your diet or your lean tissues) and use gluconeogenesis to transform them into the sugar it needs.

Yes, your body will do what it takes to get sugar. So is that addiction, or just survival?

I think we should take a lesson from nature and consider the wisdom of the body when it comes to sugar.

DOES SUGAR MAKE YOU FAT?

Science says... not really. Surprised? If you've ever read any diet or health book, you probably think I've lost my mind. But in reality, research does not back up the theory that sugar is an inherently fattening food.

In fact, studies that compare sugar to other carbohydrates show that both tend to have a similar effect on body composition. And an analysis of several sugar studies shows the same trend: sugar intake is *not* associated with obesity. Interestingly enough, one study showed that a diet high in fruit (which would be relatively high in sugar) is associated with weight *loss*.

This is not to say it's impossible to gain weight eating sugar. There is definitely some research that points to sugar being fattening under specific conditions, such as in a diet high in vegetable oils, which is (probably not by coincidence) the typical modern diet.

It's far more important to think of sugar in context of the overall diet and lifestyle, and not simply make it the scapegoat for all modern ills because it's convenient to do so.

SUGAR: NOT A DEMON (JUST A CARB)

So let's take the emotionally-charged arguments off the table and just look at the basic facts. Sugar is really just a simple carbohydrate that your body uses as glucose for energy. And while the glycemic index doesn't show the whole picture of blood sugar levels, it's interesting to note that sugar falls into the "medium-glycemic" category and raises your blood sugar *less* than foods like bread, potatoes, and white rice.

Sugar (especially in more natural forms like fruit or raw honey) can be particularly helpful if you have trouble tolerating grains and starches, because sugar is easily digested and doesn't tend to cause gut problems like starches can in sensitive individuals.

The question comes back to **energy versus nutrients**. Sugar provides energy but not always nutrients. Fruit, fruit juice, raw honey, and real maple syrup are some foods that naturally contain a balance of sugar with some nutrients.

Does this make white sugar especially bad for you? Not necessarily. White sugar is a very poor source of nutrients, obviously, but it does provide energy so it's not metabolically useless.

The key is balance. You want a diet that balances protein, fats, and carbohydrates, as well as energy and nutrients. **In this context, there is room for sugar in a healthy diet, provided it's only part of your diet and not overshadowing important nutrients you need from other foods.** So eat your fruit with some eggs or cheese, and enjoy your dessert after a balanced meal. And most importantly, listen to your body and adjust accordingly.

WATER MYTHS

Another great cultural myth is that more water is always better. There seems to be a pervasive fear that without forcing glass after glass of water down our throats, we will all suffer the terrible effects of dehydration.

We're told to always carry around a bottle of water, to drink a glass with every meal or snack, drink when you wake up and drink when you go to sleep. But we're rarely advised to do the most simple and logical thing: drink when we're thirsty.

Water clearly plays an important role in our bodies and hydration is critical for good metabolic health. But we should always be aiming for balance, not just more is better. And with water, balance is key. Hydrate the wrong way, and you can actually promote metabolic imbalances and even stress your metabolism.

This is especially true when you have low metabolic function. A slow metabolism (aka low thyroid function) typically loses electrolytes and retains water. This causes imbalances on a cellular level. This is why your individual metabolic health is a determining factor in your need for salt and water—and why listening to your body is so key for finding that balance of what your body needs on a given day.

1. COUNT ALL SOURCES OF WATER.

It seems like this would be obvious, but water is in many of the foods and beverages we consume every day anyway. But mainstream advice tells us to ignore all that and still drink no less than eight glasses of pure water per day. Some health advocates even say you shouldn't count milk or soups or other liquid-rich foods. Which, if you think about it logically, doesn't make much sense.

Your body uses all of the liquid you consume, whether it

comes in the form of fruit, milk, broth, juice or plain-Jane water. So, depending on your diet, you may not need to add several glasses of water on top of what you normally eat and drink.

2. A VARIETY OF FACTORS DETERMINE WATER NEEDS.

Just like eating a lot of water-rich foods may decrease your need for extra water, the way you live and even *where* you live can affect your hydration needs. For example, those in a cool, humid climate will likely need less water than someone living in a hot, arid region.

As with calories, a slow metabolism doesn't need as much water as a fast metabolism. You may find your thirst level increases as you nourish your metabolism and your metabolic rate increases.

Your activity level will also influence how much water you need. For instance, heavy exercisers and athletes will need a lot more water than a sedentary person (more on that in a minute).

3. BALANCE WATER WITH ELECTROLYTES

To learn about balanced rehydration, it helps to take a look at how the pros handle it.

What does the hospital do with a critically dehydrated patient? Hook them up to an IV of course. And is that IV full of plain water? Nope, it sure isn't. It is typically a saline solution (water and sodium) and sometimes glucose (sugar) is also part of the mix. Interesting, huh?

Rehydration formulas recommended by the WHO (World Health Organization) and UNICEF include sodium, potassium, and glucose in addition to water.

Why isn't plain water enough? When the body is stressed and dehydrated, it tends to waste sodium and other important electrolytes. These need to be replenished in addition to water in order to get you properly hydrated.

Sugar is also an important part of the puzzle because carbohydrates help lower stress hormones and return the body to a metabolic state that is better able to maintain a proper balance of water, sodium, and electrolytes.

THE BALANCED WAY TO REHYDRATE

If you're thirsty, then hydrate yourself with a balanced liquid. Diluted juice is a great base for a rehydration drink, and you can add a dash or two of salt to keep your sodium levels balanced. You'd be surprise how much this enhances the taste! Orange juice in particular can be an excellent liquid for rehydration. It contains potassium and magnesium, as well as natural sugars. Dilute as needed, add a little salt, and you're ready to drink!

Work on listening to your body when it comes to hydration. Notice that there are probably times of the day when you feel thirstier than others: that's the best time to drink more liquids or eat more water-heavy foods (like fruit and soup). This can be at different times for different people. Some people notice more thirst in the mornings while some notice it in the evenings.

And if you just feel a little thirsty, don't feel like you have to down a quart of liquid to quench your thirst. You may only need a few ounces. I look at hydration like I look at hunger. Have a little, and your body will let you know if it needs more. I often just drink four to eight ounces at a time. Then I wait a few minutes before seeing if my body needs more. Sometimes it does; sometimes it doesn't.

WHAT ABOUT HYDRATING DURING EXERCISE?

If you do exercise heavily or play vigorous sports, then it shouldn't be a surprise that your water needs may increase quite a bit. Providing extra hydration before, during, and after strenuous physical activity is a healthy practice. Heavy exercise will also cause you to lose electrolytes (through perspiration) and burn a lot of energy, so it's still important to practice balanced hydration by replenishing salt, minerals, and sugar as needed.

REPLACE DOGMA WITH BALANCE

While I like clearing up myths and misconceptions, health issues are not all or nothing. Salt, sugar and water aren't *always* good for you or *always* bad for you. More is not always better, but less isn't always better either. It's important to strike the balance between being too restrictive and being too passive about what you put in your body.

The point is to become aware of different aspects and potential effects of certain substances, and then becoming aware of how these different substances affect *your* body. Then you can make healthy choices based on the feedback your body is giving you, instead of following meaningless recommendations that may or may not work in your life.

Chapter 7:
Supplements
versus Superfoods

THE CULTURE OF HEALTH ENTHUSIASTS seem to endorse taking dozen of vitamins and herbal supplements every day to counterbalance nutrient deficiencies and environmental toxins. But if you're taking the wrong supplements (or simply too many of them) you may just be compounding the problem instead of making it better.

Several years ago, I was reading through a few popular health books and started taking notes on what supplements were recommended. I seemed to have almost every health problem the authors listed on their charts, so before long, I had an entire page of vitamins, minerals, and herbs to buy! This translated into roughly 40 pills every day. And taking all those capsules and tablets was not fun. Not fun at all.

Thank goodness my common sense eventually kicked in. I'm not totally against taking any supplements, but I do believe that it's important to supplement with certain principles in mind.

EAT YOUR SUPERFOODS!

A nourished metabolism does use more energy, and it also uses more nutrients. So as your energy needs go up, so do your needs for certain vitamins, minerals and other nutrients. To avoid deficiencies, it's important to supply your metabolism with the nutrients it needs, preferably through your diet.

Avoiding many supplements is possible with the addition of certain superfoods that provide specific nutrients in higher doses. Choose foods that are especially nutritious and can provide high levels of nutrients in nature's intended form:

- **MILK AND OTHER DAIRY PRODUCTS.** The higher quality, the better. Excellent for calcium intake (especially if you need to balance phosphorous intake from grains). Also contains vitamin A, vitamin K2, and B vitamins. Yogurt, kefir, and other fermented dairy are great choices if you have a sensitive digestive system.

- **BUTTER.** Butter from grass-fed cows is very nutritious and is a good source of vitamin A and vitamin K2, as well as important fatty acids like butyric acid. If you're sensitive to dairy, ghee from grass-fed cows can sometimes be better tolerated than butter, because the milk solids have been removed from ghee.

- **BUTTER OIL.** This is a concentrated form of butterfat and contains a high amount of vitamin K2, which is an important nutrient for remineralizing bones and teeth, and is also protective against heart disease.
- **FRUITS.** Excellent source for magnesium, potassium, folate, and vitamin C among other nutrients and antioxidants.
- **OYSTERS AND SHRIMP.** Contain high levels of zinc, copper, and the antioxidant mineral selenium.
- **LIVER.** Eat liver from a high quality source (such as grass-fed beef) once or twice per week for its very high vitamin A and B vitamin content.
- **COD LIVER OIL.** Excellent source of vitamins A and D. Only ½ to 1 teaspoon per day, because this oil is high in polyunsaturated fats.
- **EGG YOLKS.** Provides vitamin A, B vitamins, vitamin D, iodine, zinc, selenium and more. Eating a couple of eggs every day can really help fill up those nutrient quotas.
- **NUTRITIONAL YEAST.** Great for supplementing B vitamins, if needed.

- **REAL BONE BROTH.** Broth made with bones and joints will contain gelatin protein and calcium, as well as other important minerals.

- **BROTH FROM LEAFY GREENS.** Another way to supplement your mineral intake is to boil leafy greens (like kale and spinach) and then use the plain broth for drinking or cooking. This extracts the nutrients from the greens, and leaves indigestible materials behind.

TIPS FOR USING SUPPLEMENTS WISELY

If you feel your diet is lacking in certain nutrients, and you decide to try supplementing, it's okay to try adding a few key supplements to your daily routine. In fact, some of the herbal remedies and nutrients I've mentioned in this book can be very helpful as supplements. It's all about approaching them with some wisdom and balance. Here are a few helpful principles you can follow to minimize potential problems:

- **PILLS DON'T REPLACE A NUTRIENT-DENSE DIET.** Nutrients from food are part of a package deal of synergistic co-factors that complement absorption and improve usability. And supplement manufacturers are slow to catch up with nature. Every year, researchers find more cofactors present in real foods that enhance how our bodies use specific nutrients. We have barely scratched the surface! So whenever possible, get your nutrients from food for the best results.

- **MORE IS NOT ALWAYS BETTER.** Only use supplements when there is a genuine need. The supplement industry is not well regulated, and products are not always pure. The fewer supplements you use, the less potential there is for negative reactions.

- **NEVER JUMP RIGHT INTO MEGA-DOSING WITH ANY NUTRIENT.** The best way to avoid possible side effects and to gauge how your body reacts to specific nutrients is to start small and work your way up as needed. Then you can determine the dose that's right for your body. (Sometimes less is more.)

- **INTRODUCE ONE SUPPLEMENT AT A TIME.** If you want to know what works and what doesn't, you can't start taking half a dozen supplements at once and expect to be able to interpret the results clearly. A good rule of thumb would be to give each new supplement or dosage a two to four week trial run before trying anything else.

- **CHECK THE INGREDIENTS.** Supplements are often loaded with additives, many of which are potentially irritating to the digestive tract. Powder or liquid forms often contain fewer or even no additives. Pills made with simple gelatin capsules or softgels are usually the next best thing. Avoid tablets when possible, as they contain binders that may irritate your digestive system.

- **WATCH OUT FOR COMBINATION FORMULAS.** Beware of supplements that throw in a variety of vitamins, minerals, and herbs to form a fancy complex. Some of these are beneficial, but most are using the complex as a way to "water down" more expensive ingredients with cheap fillers. Plus, if you have an adverse reaction, it will be difficult to tell which ingredient is causing the problem.

- **TAKE SUPPLEMENTS WITH MEALS.** Unless it is otherwise indicated, most supplements should be taken with a full meal. This gets nutrients packaged together with fat, protein, carbohydrates, and other co-factors that will enhance absorption.

Chapter 8:
Why You Need Better Sleep and How to Get It

I WOKE UP... AGAIN. It was the third time that night, and each time it took me an hour or more to fall back asleep. I calculated the total number of hours I could sleep before I had to get up the next morning. Four. The answer was four. Even if I slept through the rest of the night I was only getting four hours of sleep. And I cried.

This used to be me, almost every single night. Living without sleep is a nightmare, and it tends to be a vicious cycle that perpetuates itself through elevated stress hormones and anxiety. Let's put a stop to that cycle and start getting some rest!

PUTTING SLEEP ON A PEDESTAL

I think most of us know that we feel better when we get a good night's sleep. But with today's busy schedules, making sleep a priority just doesn't happen as much as it should. Sometimes it's just easier to ignore your chronic sleep deprivation, and instead try to address your health problems with food and supplements; but this will only get you so far.

If you don't get enough quality sleep, healthy habits in other areas will have minimal results. Even the healthiest food is not going to solve your health problems if you don't make sleep a priority. It's like turning a light on in the bathroom when you're trying to find something in a dark basement. No matter how bright that light is, it's not where you need it.

Quality sleep has a profound impact on your metabolic health. It affects your moods, your cognitive ability, your blood sugar, your stress hormone levels, and so much more. If you haven't been making time for sleep, it's time to make a change.

SLEEP DEPRIVATION STRESSES YOUR METABOLISM

Lack of sleep is a direct stress on the body. Sleep studies show that even one night of poor sleep can elevate your cortisol levels the next day. Imagine what happens when you sleep poorly almost every night! It's a recipe for chronically high stress hormones.

And right along with raising your stress hormone levels, research shows that poor quality sleep also interferes with insulin sensitivity. That same one night of bad sleep can actually prevent your body from being able to balance your blood sugar the next day! In the long run, poor sleep habits can increase your risk for diabetes.

The trouble doesn't end there. Not getting enough sleep is also associated with poor brain function, increased anxiety, low moods, depression, and increased risk of stroke.

Not a pretty picture, is it? But the good news is that turning your sleep habits around can potentially turn your health around as well.

HOW MUCH SLEEP DO YOU NEED?

Based on research connecting sleep with metabolic health issues, **most experts recommend *at least* seven hours of quality, uninterrupted sleep every night.** This is the *bare minimum* you should be aiming for on a daily basis. But if you're exhausted, stressed, and in poor metabolic health, you may need extra sleep as your body heals. In my experience, many people benefit from sleeping no less than eight to ten hours on most nights when they first start working on their metabolic health. This may be needed for several weeks or even months as their body heals.

The extra rest can be an important key for healing by leaps and bounds. If you don't get enough sleep and have been struggling to show improvements in biofeedback, then prioritizing sleep may help you finally turn your health around. Even when your metabolic health is great, in times of stress, it's a good idea to prioritize sleep more than you normally would. This can help counteract the negative effects of stress and help you bounce back faster when things get back to normal.

Depending on your schedule and your life situation (if you have young children, for example), it may be difficult to make enough time for sleep. I urge you to do what you can to squeeze in a few extra hours every week if at all possible. Go to bed an hour early some nights, sleep in on the weekends, or catch a nap now and then. Every little bit helps, and once you start feeling more rested, you may be surprised how much more focus and energy you can bring to your life. You may actually get *more* done when you schedule more time for sleep!

"What if Sleep Makes Me Tired?"

I find this happens in more extreme cases of exhaustion. If you usually sleep four to six hours a night and suddenly you start sleeping for eight hours or more, you may find yourself needing more sleep than ever! This was the case for me in the beginning, and sometimes it felt like I could never get enough sleep.

This happens when your sleep deprivation is actually fueling your energy levels by keeping your stress hormones unnaturally propped up. When you've been doing this for a long time and you suddenly start sleeping more, the lack of stress hormones may uncover your underlying fatigue. It's really important to push past this and give your body the rest it needs to heal, rather than going back to old habits to self-medicate and feel better temporarily.

If this is the case for you, it helps to remember this is temporary and just part of the healing process. As your body recovers and gets some much-needed rest, your energy levels will slowly return to normal. How quickly this happens usually depends on how long you've been sleep deprived. If you've spent years with sleep deprivation, don't expect to bounce back in a couple of weeks! Give your body some time to heal, and you will reap the reward of feeling more rested and energetic as time goes on.

BUILD AN ENVIRONMENT FOR SLEEP

If you have a hard time sleeping, a few small adjustments can make a big difference. Set the stage for sleep, and it may come more easily than you think.

GET COMFORTABLE. Make sure your bed, pillows, lighting, and room temperature are all conducive to sleep. Nothing will kill your sleep like a bright porch light, a lumpy mattress, or a stifling hot room.

THE LAST HOUR BEFORE BED IS RESERVED FOR RELAXATION. Don't run around finishing up chores or projects right before bedtime—do something restful and calming instead. It might be a warm bath in Epsom salts, which contain magnesium that can promote sleep. Or try reading a good book or listening to some calming music. Watching television or drinking a glass of wine, although not exactly ideal, may also help you unwind; but I'd recommend trying some other ideas as well. Don't watch anything too stimulating (sorry action fans!) or drink too much alcohol before bed, which can put you to sleep at first, but can also cause blood sugar to drop in the middle of the night which will wake you back up!

DIM THE LIGHTS. Darkness signals the body it's time to rest. So turn off the bright lights and spend that time before bed with just enough light to enjoy your restful activities. Warm, yellow light is more sleep-friendly than bright, blue lighting.

WATCH YOUR CAFFEINE INTAKE. Avoid caffeine during the last several hours of the day. Sensitive individuals may need to stay away from caffeine anytime after noon, or may need to cut it out altogether to really get results. This varies person to person, so make sure to listen to your body on this one.

NAP IF YOU NEED TO, BUT NOT TOO MUCH. Limit daytime naps to less than an hour, and take a nap before 4:00 in the afternoon if possible. You want to condition your body to sleep mainly at night. If napping during the day doesn't interfere with your sleep at night, that probably means you're in need of the extra rest, and you can continue napping as needed. If you notice your naps start interfering with your sleep, you probably need to limit the time you spend napping. Power naps (less than 30 minutes long) can sometimes help you feel rested and more focused without interfering with nighttime sleep.

BEDTIME SNACKS FOR BETTER SLEEP

Eating the right snack before bed can lower your stress hormones and help you fall asleep. This will also keep your blood sugar levels from plummeting too low during the night, causing your stress hormones to rise and waking you up. If you do wake up in the middle of the night and have trouble falling back asleep, a small snack can often help get you back to sleep quickly.

A stress-reducing snack will include some carbohydrates, fats, and protein. The combination is satisfying and provides the body with the different fuels and rebuilding materials it needs to get through the night without raising stress hormones to make up for what's missing. Including something with a little salt and gelatin can be especially helpful. Salt helps lower stress hormones, and the glycine in gelatin will raise your levels of the amino acid GABA, which is known for its calming effect.

Here are a few examples of balanced bedtime nibbles:

- Hot chocolate made with milk, maple syrup, a scoop of gelatin protein, and a dash of salt.
- Fruit and cheese.
- Real broth with gelatin and salt, with a side of rice or dried fruit.

- A small bowl of ice cream or a piece of cheesecake, with salted macadamia nuts or cheese on the side.

HERBAL REMEDIES FOR BETTER SLEEP

Sometimes we need a little extra support helping us get to sleep and stay asleep, especially in the beginning when we're still working on balancing all those good habits for reducing stress. Herbal remedies are a gentle way to nudge the body into the habit of better sleep. You can have a cup of herbal tea before bed to help you wind down. You can also try herbal tinctures or capsules if you're not a fan of tea. Here are some beneficial herbs before sleep:

- Valerian
- Chamomile
- Lemon balm (Melissa)
- Magnolia bark

Essential oils can also be used to reduce stress and help you sleep. Apply a few drops with a little carrier oil (like coconut oil) to the wrists, ankles, and feet before bed. Or apply to a handkerchief and slip it into your pillowcase to help you fall asleep. Some of the best essential oils for sleep include to following:

- Lavender
- Cedarwood
- Orange
- Chamomile

DON'T STRESS ABOUT SLEEP!

Lack of sleep can cause a vicious cycle. We can't sleep, so we stress about not being able to sleep; and the stress makes it even harder to sleep! Although sleeping enough is important, it's not worth stressing over. So if you're having trouble sleeping, here's some tips on handling it with the right perspective:

DON'T KEEP A CLOCK IN VIEW OF THE BED. First, digital clocks can disrupt your circadian rhythms by exposing you to unnatural light at night. Second, if you check the clock every time you wake up and keep track of how long it's taking you to fall back asleep, it usually only serves to increase your stress and make it even *harder* to fall asleep!

IF YOU HAVE TO GET UP, KEEP THE LIGHTS LOW. Whether it's a trip to the bathroom, or a visit to the kitchen to make a bedtime snack, use the lowest light setting possible. Bright lights signal your body that it's time to wake up—not what you want to do in the middle of the night!

REMEMBER THAT IT'S *OKAY* TO WAKE UP AT NIGHT. It's normal to wake during light sleep occasionally during the night. In fact, most of us do it without even noticing it because we slip back into a deep sleep so quickly. So simply waking up during the night is no cause for panic. Just take a deep breath, remind yourself that this is normal, and get comfortable.

STAY CALM. If you wake up at night, don't take it as an opportunity to mentally plan your next grocery run, worry about asking your boss for a raise, or think about what you should have said to your mother-in-law when she commented about the weird smell in your kitchen yesterday. Now is not the time to think about things that make your heart race!

Instead, remind yourself that this is the time for rest and sleep, and there will be plenty of time tomorrow to deal with what needs to be done. I've often found that once I've slept on things, they never seem like a big deal the next day—even though I was worrying and stressing about them at 3:00 in the morning!

GIVE IT TIME. Better sleep will come with time and practice. It sounds funny, but we really do have to practice at sleep. Every day you make a positive change in your sleep habits, the more you build healthy sleep patterns. Eventually, good sleep will come to you naturally. But at first, it will seem a lot like taking two steps forward and one step back. You might get a great night's sleep one night, only to not have another one for two weeks! But as time goes on, you should see more good nights than bad nights; and eventually, a bad night's sleep will be a rarity.

It really helps to remember this is all *normal*. As you develop healthy habits and eat well, it will get easier and easier to fall asleep and stay asleep. Pretty soon you won't even have to think about it!

Chapter 9: Smart and Balanced Exercise

Almost everyone would love an excuse *not* to exercise—probably because exercise has become a rather tortured experience in modern culture. Most noticeably, long-distance running and other endurance exercises have become in vogue during the last few decades, which leads many to believe if you aren't running, biking, spinning, or speed-walking for at least an hour every day, you're just not doing enough to make a difference.

This is a flat-out misconception, and it generally leads to doing far too much exercise—or giving up and doing none at all. But like everything else we've discussed so far, balance is the key to using exercise to support your metabolism and improve your health.

You don't have to spend hours and hours every week at the gym in order to reap the benefits of exercise. In fact, *overdoing* exercise is one of the top metabolic stressors of the modern age—right up there with not eating well and not getting enough quality sleep. Put all three of those together, and you've got the recipe for a metabolic disaster.

WHY MOVEMENT IS MORE IMPORTANT THAN EXERCISE

When someone talks about being more active, it's natural to assume they mean making time for the gym. But simply "exercising" may not be the most important part of being active. Making movement part of your everyday lifestyle may be crucial to improving your health.

Research indicates that time spent sitting down (such as at the computer, in front of the TV, or in the car) directly correlates with reduced longevity, poor insulin sensitivity, heart disease and more.

Those who spend more time sitting down versus being up and about are more likely to experience health problems and possibly an earlier death. This is independent of exercise habits, meaning those who sit the most have the most health issues, even if they "exercise" regularly.

A New Take on "Sedentary"

The problem begins with how we define being sedentary versus being active. Most people focus on how much and how often you participate in a particular form of exercise: running, going to the gym, popping in a workout DVD, etc. If you work out for 30-60 minutes, 3-5 times per week, most health professionals would consider you an active person—even if all you do the rest of the time is sit in the car, at the computer, or in front of the television.

And the person who never does any formal exercise, but walks to work, gardens regularly and plays dodge ball with the kids outside every evening, may not be considered active at all because they don't log the hours at the gym or on a treadmill.

So it really comes down to common sense when defining whether you're active or sedentary. It also requires some self-awareness, because you have to be honest about the amount of activity you really do in a day. It may be a lot less than you think!

Including a little more activity throughout your day can be as simple as taking a five-minute break from the desk at work every hour or two, and switching to an activity that gets your body moving for a few minutes. Take a walk, do some housework, or do a few stretches or body-weight exercises.

If you don't know whether you're active or not, a pedometer can be a handy gadget for gauging how much you really move throughout the day, especially if you have a desk job or tend to be sitting down all the time. It will measure your daily activity, and the pedometer doesn't lie!

ENDURANCE EXERCISE = STRESS

Long sessions of endurance exercise (also known as cardio or aerobic exercise) requires the body to switch fuel sources so it can burn protein and fat for energy. This causes the release of stress hormones like cortisol and adrenaline. By long sessions, I mean doing moderate to intense activity for more than an hour at a time. Shorter bursts of activity can be beneficial (more on that in a bit), but when you take it too far and start trying to run a marathon every week, you could be putting too much strain on the body.

When you're doing endurance exercise on a regular basis (especially when you're not eating and sleeping enough to support the activity), this can lead to chronically high stress hormone levels. Chronic over-exercising tends to be catabolic (breaks down lean tissue like muscles) and often leads to a low resting pulse, which is a sign of a slow metabolic rate.

Emerging research reveals that lifelong endurance exercise enthusiasts (like marathon runners) may actually have a *higher* rate of heart problems. This is the opposite of what we've heard for years about aerobic exercise ("It's so good for your heart!"), but it actually make sense from a metabolic perspective. If heavy endurance activity is metabolically suppressive, it can lead to disorders like heart disease and diabetes, conditions linked to a low metabolic rate.

Heavy exercising has also been connected to other symptoms of a stressed metabolism, such as:

- Poor immune system function
- Fatigue and exhaustion
- Sleep disturbances
- Mood problems

If you have a stressed metabolism, and you've been doing a lot of endurance exercise, it may be time to rethink your workout routine. It's time to stop doing *more* exercise and start doing *smart* exercise.

SMART EXERCISE KEY #1: SUPPORT EXERCISE WITH YOUR LIFESTYLE

This means eating and sleeping to support your activity level. If you exercise more, you need to eat more, especially protein and carbohydrates to support your energy needs and muscle activity. You also need to be sleeping well to support regular exercise. If you're only sleeping five hours every night and running for an hour every day, you're on the fast path to exhaustion. **If you want to be fit, you first need to be rested.**

If you're severely exhausted and calorie-deprived, it might help to take a hiatus from exercising. You're not going to lose your edge if you set aside two to three weeks for resting and rebuilding. From there, you can start slowly, if needed, and work your way up to a balanced exercise routine.

If you don't do much exercise, then it's also a good idea to work your way up slowly. No need for boot-camp style torture sessions! To get in shape and get healthy, your body and your muscles need to adapt gradually to being more active. Supported by a healthy diet and good sleep habits, becoming more active will come more naturally over time. It's consistency that matters.

SMART EXERCISE KEY #2: EXERCISE FOR YOUR METABOLISM

If your metabolism is stressed, now is not the time to sign up for marathon training. The goal isn't being sedentary, of course, but you want to exercise in moderation, especially while you work toward lowering stress hormone levels. Relaxing walks outdoors can keep you active without causing a lot of stress. In fact, research shows that walking in nature actually *lowers* your cortisol levels! You can also add in a couple of weekly sessions of strength training, swimming, yoga, or similar activities. These keep your muscles healthy and active, but don't tend to cause metabolic stress if done in moderation (about 20-30 minutes per session).

SMART EXERCISE KEY #3: PAY ATTENTION TO BIOFEEDBACK

How do you feel after exercise? If you're doing the right exercise for your current metabolic state, you should feel pleasantly energized after exercise. What you should NOT feel is:

- Exhausted, tense, and in too much pain to get through normal tasks for the rest of the day.
- An incredible burst of energy and excitement, followed by a severe energy crash within a couple of hours.

You want your exercise routine to *add* to your life, not detract from it or leave you feeling too fatigued to live it. If that happens consistently, you might want to try cutting back on the duration or frequency of your workouts.

SMART EXERCISE KEY #4: DO WHAT YOU LOVE!

Whatever exercise you love and enjoy doing is the right exercise for you. It doesn't matter if it's kick-boxing, surfing, swimming, gardening, tai chi, yoga, weight lifting, walking, dancing, or any other activity that gets your body moving.

Love running, biking, and other aerobic activities? You don't necessarily have to give them up to get healthy! If you have signs of a stressed metabolism, you may have to cut down on the duration or frequency of your workouts, at least temporarily. But it's not an all or nothing venture.

Figure out the right balance that allows you to do the activity you love without negatively impacting your metabolic health. This may mean shorter runs or a fewer miles on the bike every week, or it may mean putting more emphasis on diet and sleep in order to support additional activity. **Learn to be aware of how exercise affects your body, so you can make choices that enhance your metabolic health.**

Certain types of exercise may offer specific benefits; but in the end, it's all about what fits best with *your* life, *your* metabolism, and *your* personality.

HIIT: GET THE MOST OUT OF A SHORT WORKOUT

If you don't have time to exercise—or if you love cardio and don't want to give it up altogether—you might want to think about switching to HIIT (High Intensity Interval Training).

The basic idea of HIIT is that you exercise in short bursts of intense activity for up to 60 seconds at a time. In between bursts, your activity level should be easy or moderate, and long enough for you to catch your breath. Sessions are shorter than traditional aerobic workouts, generally lasting only about 10-20 minutes, with a few minutes to warm up before and cool down after. That means your total workout time for an HIIT workout will usually be about 20-30 minutes. The shortened length keeps these workouts from shifting into the endurance phase where the body has to burn alternative fuel sources with stress hormones, but the intensity still gives your heart and your muscles a great workout.

The principles of HIIT can be incorporated into whatever workout system you prefer. You can do HIIT while walking, running, swimming, jumping on a trampoline, lifting weights, riding a bike, or jumping rope. Basically, you can do HIIT with whatever equipment you already have, or even with no equipment at all.

For example, during a leisurely stroll or bike ride, throw in a few 30-60 second bursts of intense activity with recovery periods in between. So if you're walking, break into a full run for about 60 seconds and then slow back down to an easy walk until you catch your breath. You can start with about one to two intervals per workout, and work your way up to three to six intervals per workout over a period of weeks.

Research has revealed a few key metabolic benefits of HIIT:

- Improvements in heart health,
- Improved blood-sugar levels and insulin sensitivity,
- Increased fat loss compared to aerobic exercise.

These specific benefits speak volumes about how HIIT impacts your health at a metabolic level. It's the perfect example of how exercising *smarter*—instead of just exercising *more*—can improve your metabolic health.

HOW BUILDING YOUR MUSCLES NOURISHES YOUR METABOLISM

I won't repeat the tired mantra that muscle burns more calories than fat—although it's technically true—as if that's the *only* reason building muscle is good for you. The science behind strength training is much more interesting than mere calorie expenditure.

Research has shown that muscle-building exercise has specific health benefits which indicate a positive change in the underlying metabolism:

- **STRENGTH TRAINING IMPROVES INSULIN SENSITIVITY.** Research demonstrates that weight-bearing exercise has a positive effect on insulin sensitivity, which can help keep your blood-sugar levels steady.

- **WEIGHT-BEARING EXERCISE STRENGTHENS YOUR BONES AND JOINTS.** There have been numerous studies that show strength training exercises improve bone health and increase bone density.

- **BUILDING YOUR MUSCLES MAY ALSO BUILD YOUR BRAIN.** Research indicates that resistance training exercises can actually improve cognitive functions like memory, attention, and processing speed.

- **RESISTANCE EXERCISE CAN IMPROVE YOUR MOOD.** Both anxiety and depression have been shown to improve with resistance training. Even chronic fatigue can be relieved with strength training.

How often should you do strength training exercises? A basic formula is 2-3 times per week for 30-45 minutes (depending on your metabolic health). But I definitely encourage you to find a workout routine that feels good for you and fits into your life. Aim to build up strength and endurance over time. You can do this through weight lifting, yoga, or just simple bodyweight exercises. Give yourself plenty of recovery time in between workouts (at least one full day).

EXERCISE FOR THE EXHAUSTED

If you are stressed, exhausted, sick, and have a low body temperature, you have to be choosy about your exercise. That means exercising smarter, not more. If you're having a hard time eating or sleeping enough to support a moderate activity level, it may be best to limit yourself to a few weekly walks at first. When you feel well enough, add in one to two weekly sessions of strength training or yoga to improve your muscle strength. Increase your activity level gradually as you make positive changes in stress reduction, diet, and sleep habits.

Chapter 10:
Biofeedback: It's What Your Body Has to Say

HOW DO YOU KNOW if a suggestion is working for you? Listen to your body! Your body is actually pretty good at telling you what works and what doesn't, but most of us have forgotten how to listen to it.

Biofeedback is one of the most important tools you can use to determine what your body needs and what it thrives on. Your body can tell you if your diet, exercise plan, or lifestyle needs to be tweaked to give you that metabolic boost you need. It can also give you concrete evidence that you are making progress in your health efforts, which can give you the patience and encouragement you need to make a continued effort toward improving your health.

Let's discuss some of the easiest ways you can listen to what your body is telling you and keep track of your metabolic improvements:

BODY TEMPERATURE

Taking your temperature is one of the best ways to measure how your metabolism is functioning. Basically, a higher temperature is a reflection of a higher metabolism, and a lower body temperature reflects a lower metabolism.

How and When to Take Your Body Temperature

IN THE MORNING:

- Take your underarm temperature in the morning before rising.
- It should be somewhere between 97.8 and 98.6 degrees Fahrenheit. A temperature lower than 97.8 could indicate a lower than optimal metabolism.
- Higher is not always better, though. A temperature higher than 98.6 may indicate high stress hormones.
- Menstruating women may experience a slightly higher temperature during the second half of their cycle, so a higher reading during this time is normal.
- Thermometers specially made for taking your underarm

temperature can be helpful.

- Leaving the thermometer under your arm for a few extra minutes may give you a more accurate reading.

AFTER BREAKFAST:

- About 30-60 minutes after you've eaten breakfast, take your temperature again, just not after a hot shower or being too active as these can alter your reading.
- After eating, your temperature should be higher than your first reading (due to the thermogenic effects of food).
- If your temperature goes *down* after eating, it may be a sign that your stress hormones are too high. High stress hormones can cause your body temperature to be high upon waking, but then eating will lower your stress hormones and bring your temperature back down.
- The "after-breakfast" test is the best way to see if stress hormones are falsely propping up your waking temperature.

AT MID-AFTERNOON:

- Sometime between about 2:00 and 4:00 PM in the afternoon, check your temperature again.
- It should be in the 97.8–98.6 range, similar to your waking temperature or somewhat higher. (Being active during the day can bring your temperature up slightly.)

NOTE: Don't worry! You don't have to take your temperature three times a day, every day, for the rest of your life. Instead, track your temperature for a few days to get an average. Repeat this procedure every few weeks to gauge your progress, or whenever you feel off and want to get a baseline on your metabolism.

HEART RATE (PULSE)

Similar to body temperature, a low pulse rate can indicate low metabolic function. The ideal range is somewhere between about 75–85 beats per minute (bpm). You can check your pulse with an oximeter or a stopwatch at the same times you check your basal temperature (upon waking, after breakfast, and in the afternoon).

SKIN, HAIR AND NAILS

Changes in your skin, hair, and nails are an important source of biofeedback. Although they seem like surface issues, by looking at what's happening on the outside of our bodies, we get some clues about what's happening on the inside, too. You see, your skin cells are constantly being replaced. And your hair and nails are constantly being built so they can continue to grow. If your metabolism isn't functioning properly, these simple systems don't work efficiently. Problems with skin, hair, and nails quickly start to crop up.

NOURISHED SKIN:

- Soft, smooth, and dewy
- Balanced oil production
- Fewer, smaller blemishes
- Thick, elastic, and "bounces back"
- Even toned, little redness

STRESSED SKIN:

- Dry, flaky
- Very oily or greasy
- Acne and/or cysts
- Thin, papery, low-elasticity
- Redness, inflammation

NOURISHED HAIR:

- Thick, few thin spots
- Bright and deep color
- Shiny, strong
- Normal oil production

STRESSED HAIR:

- Thinning
- Dull and faded
- Dry, brittle
- Overly oily

NOURISHED NAILS:

- Strong, not very bendable
- Long, not prone to cracking

STRESSED NAILS:

- Weak and bendable
- Short due to cracking and peeling

Keep in mind, a nourished metabolism may not cause all your hair to grow back if you're balding, or color your hair if you're graying. But there's no doubt that a balanced, nutrient-dense diet supports the health of your hair, skin, and nails. It may take time for these metabolic improvements to show up; but over a period of weeks, you should be able to tell if things are moving in a positive direction.

SLEEP PATTERNS

Sleep can tell you a lot about your metabolic health. It's hard to sleep well when your stress hormones are chronically high, and sleep problems tend to get progressively worse if you don't address the underlying issues.

Depending on a lot of factors, a good night's sleep should be about seven to nine hours of relatively unbroken sleep. If you do wake once or twice, which is normal to some degree, you find it easy to fall back asleep within a few minutes.

If your stress hormones are high, a few sleep problems will start to appear, such as:

- Difficulty falling asleep,
- Waking frequently during the night,
- Waking in the early morning (2:00–4:00 am) and not being able to fall back asleep,
- Waking up early even though you're only getting five to seven hours of sleep.

These are signs of high stress hormones. If you can catch these patterns when they first start, it's much easier to get your sleep back on track. (Refer to Chapter 8 for more tips on sleep.)

ENERGY AND MOOD

Extreme moods and energy levels on either end of the spectrum are signs of a stressed metabolism. Feeling too tired or even too wired is a sign of imbalance.

Ideally, your energy levels should be mostly consistent throughout the day. Sure, you'll have natural highs and lows, but you shouldn't feel like you're constantly alternating between huge bursts of energy and crippling fatigue.

Similarly, mood swings (like going from laughing to angry to weeping) also indicate a stressed metabolism. Now, you're not looking to be an emotional automaton; but you do want a degree of balance and resilience when it comes to your day-to-day moods. Sad things will make you sad–but not leave you severely depressed. And irritating things might get on your nerves, but they shouldn't leave you raging over every little inconvenience.

We're all human and life will always have its ups and downs, so it's important to keep a balanced perspective. Don't get too caught up in blaming every negative emotion on your metabolic health. But watching the overall trend of your moods and energy levels can be a very helpful form of biofeedback.

DIGESTION

Your digestion can definitely clue you in about your current metabolic state. When your body is balanced, digestion is a behind-the-scenes task. It works efficiently without you ever thinking about it. Bowel movements should be quick, easy, and regular (usually every day about the same time).

Indigestion, constipation, diarrhea, or IBS can be signs of a low metabolism, high stress hormones, and other imbalances. High stress hormones divert blood flow away from your digestive system and also shut down your immune system, which can lead to poor digestion and bacterial imbalances in your gut. Constipation can also be a sign of low magnesium levels.

Indigestion, bloating, and discomfort directly after a meal may signal that what you're eating doesn't agree with your body. This is more common in a low metabolic state, when inflammation and autoimmunity are often present and can cause food sensitivities. As you heal your metabolism, you can typically handle a wider variety of foods; but in the beginning, it may help to reduce potentially irritating foods. Instead, focus on foods that provide nutrients and energy in an easy-to-digest form, like those we talked about in Chapter 4.

BIOFEEDBACK IN PERSPECTIVE

Biofeedback is a useful tool that can help you keep track of your progress or see where your habits are holding you back. But remember to keep a balanced perspective about biofeedback. Don't let yourself get too tangled up in measuring and weighing every single factor. Remember: stress is the enemy of metabolic health!

Chapter 11:
Metabolism and Weight

THE DIET INDUSTRY HAS MONOPOLIZED the word metabolism to the degree that it begins to seem like metabolism is just about what we weigh. As we've discussed throughout this book, your metabolism is actually a reflection of how your body functions and uses energy in a myriad of ways. It relates to your moods, your sleep, your digestion, your energy levels, and much more.

Improving your metabolic health is about so much more than weight; yet in our size-conscious society, it's impossible to separate the two. The problem is that when you're primarily focused on getting to a goal weight, your metabolic health often takes the back seat to a number on the scale and suffers in the long run.

Many of the schemes that promise metabolic health are really thinly veiled attempts to market a program for obtaining six-pack abs or the body of a bikini model. And most of them are merely low-calorie diets or intense exercise regimens in disguise. These are the very behaviors that can raise your stress hormone levels and wreck your metabolic health! Yet people fall for these claims over and over, believing that weight loss automatically equals a healthy metabolism.

A NOURISHED METABOLISM IS NOT A NUMBER ON A SCALE

The truth is, a healthy metabolism has little to do with your weight. What it does have to do with is your biofeedback, like a normal body temperature, healthy skin and hair, steady energy levels, good digestive health, and resilient moods.

People can be metabolically healthy at a variety of weights. A healthy metabolism does not automatically make you thin, and especially not as thin as Hollywood standards might dictate. Studies demonstrate that overweight individuals can achieve improvements in metabolic health through *lifestyle changes* alone, even *without any change in weight.*

The point is to **prioritize your metabolic health and quality of life** *first*, and allow your weight to be a secondary consideration. This means that you *never* sacrifice the first two things in order to achieve a certain weight.

WHAT IS YOUR IDEAL WEIGHT?

Let's get clear on this from the start: your ideal weight is not the weight of the film star on television, the model on the cover of a magazine, your workout buddy at the gym, your neighbor, your sister, or anyone else who isn't *you*.

Your ideal weight is not some random number on a chart. It's not what you weighed in high school. And it's not what you weighed after you did the grapefruit diet, the egg diet, or any other fad diet.

Your ideal weight should be a side effect of doing all of the things that nourish your metabolism (like eating and sleeping well, minimizing stress, and being active). **Your ideal weight is unique to *your* body, *your* health, *your* personality, and *your* lifestyle.**

If the ideal weight at which your metabolism functions best doesn't match the ideal weight you have in your head, then it may be time for a little perspective and honesty. Figure out the real reasons you're trying to reach a certain number on the scale, and then decide whether those reasons add to the quality of your life or take away from it.

MANAGING WEIGHT WITHOUT STRESSING YOUR METABOLISM

While I strongly encourage you to make your weight a secondary priority next to nourishing your metabolism, that doesn't mean you can't consider your weight at all. You just have to consider it from a balanced perspective that doesn't reduce your body to a number on a scale or your metabolism to a number of calories-in versus calories-out.

Here are some tips on keeping a balanced perspective and managing your weight the genuinely healthy way:

1. LOVE AND ACCEPT YOUR BODY RIGHT NOW.

It sounds trite, but it's probably more important than you realize. If you want to lose weight, it's not going to happen overnight. And even if you do reach your desired weight, it's not going to magically get rid of all your imperfections. So *right now* is the time to start loving your body and treating it with respect. That means appreciating the uniqueness of your individual body. It means wearing clothes that fit correctly and make you feel great wearing them. It means never making ugly comments about your imperfections. Loving your body doesn't mean giving up any goals for improvement, but it does mean simply developing a more positive and respectful attitude about yourself and your body.

2. NOURISH YOUR METABOLISM FIRST.

Weight loss needs to be on the back burner if you have a low body temperature, poor digestion, fatigue, poor quality sleep, and other signs of a stressed metabolism. Work on the basics of nourishing your metabolism *before* putting too much focus on weight loss. For some, weight loss may occur as a natural side effect of a nourished metabolism. In any case, it's important for you to let your body accomplish some healing first.

3. BE PATIENT AND MAKE SMALL CHANGES OVER TIME.

Just like with healing your metabolism, real change in body composition takes time and patience. It takes having a long-term perspective, because a series of small, consistent changes is what makes a *real* difference—not another fad diet that promises you'll drop two dress sizes in two weeks. The body *resists* dramatic shifts in weight. It's better to work gradually for a change that lasts a lifetime, than to exhaust yourself trying to lose a few pounds that will pop right back on the minute you're too tired to keep going.

4. BE CONSISTENT AND FOLLOW A ROUTINE.

Healthy changes are much easier to make when we make them a habit. Eat at regular times, make activity part of your lifestyle, and plan your grocery list enough to make sure you have healthy food on hand (at least most of the time). Now, any changes you make should be based on what works uniquely for *you*—which is why I don't lay out a specific meal plan or exercise plan in this book. You have to get to know yourself and your body well enough to know what fits in your life and what doesn't. That may take a while at first if you're used to following someone else's plan for you. But once you get into your own groove, it's amazing how easy it is to do what's healthy for your body.

5. BE REALISTIC ABOUT YOUR GOALS.

It's important to take a step back and understand *why* you have a particular goal weight in mind. If you're choosing a goal weight based on unrealistic ideas about what your body should look like, you're going to have a difficult time staying physically and mentally healthy trying to reach that weight. Everyone's body is different, and that's the way it's supposed to be! Honor the unique individuality of your body and don't try to make it something it's not.

6. PAY ATTENTION TO INCHES, NOT POUNDS.

The scale is deceiving. It can't accurately measure whether you're losing fat, muscle, bone mass, or just water weight. It can make you think you're gaining fat when you're really gaining muscle, or it can trick you into thinking you're losing fat when really you just lost water. If you want a long-term perspective about losing weight, you aren't going to get it by hopping on the scale every day. A better way to gauge your progress is to use a measuring tape or even just a pair of pants. Measuring your waistline (and your hips, if you're a woman) once or twice per week can give you an idea of where you're going, as can your favorite pair of jeans if they're getting tighter or looser.

Keep in mind that healthy habits often get more nutrition into your bones and muscles. This lean mass weighs more than fat, and will show up on the scale *but not on your waistline.* I've heard from many women who started eating more nourishing food and gained five pounds, but their pant size stayed the same—some even had to go buy smaller pants! Looking at inches, not pounds, will give you a better idea of your true body composition.

A balanced perspective, a good dose of patience, and listening to biofeedback will help you manage your weight while keeping your metabolism healthy. But no matter what your goals are or how you plan to get there, the most important thing you can remember is this:

There is never, ever a good reason to sacrifice your health for a number on a scale.

Final Thoughts from Elizabeth

I HOPE YOU'VE BEEN ABLE TO PICK UP some helpful ideas about how to optimize your metabolic health and improve your life. Before I wrap this up, I wanted to share a few more thoughts with you.

KEEP PERSPECTIVE

Improving your health doesn't happen overnight, but I can attest to it that it is a rewarding journey. Remember that eating and living well takes practice, just like learning to swim or mastering smart phone technology. (I still don't know what some of those icons do!) It's something that comes with time and experience, and that's part of the fun. You'll always be learning more about yourself and your body, and every day is another chance to put that knowledge to good use.

ALLOW FOR TRANSITION

If you've been eating a strict diet and are ready to start being more flexible, make the transition slowly. Don't go from eating a low-carb diet to eating tons of pasta. This is not about swinging from one extreme to another! If you feel like you need to make big changes to your diet, make them slowly and give your body time to adapt to the new change. Doing this will prevent a lot of discomfort and negative side effects associated with swinging drastically from one type of diet to another.

PUT A FEW HEALTHY HABITS ON "AUTOPILOT"

The hardest part about making healthy choices is that there are so many to make! Every day we have endless opportunities to decide whether to eat this or that, take the stairs or the elevator, go to sleep early or watch one more episode of our favorite sitcom. Put a few of these choices on autopilot, and it can be much less overwhelming! For instance, I eat the same thing for breakfast almost every morning: my favorite coffee smoothie with real milk, gelatin protein, and natural sweetener. It's the same basic recipe every day so I don't even have to think about it. That's one less decision I have to worry about every day! Now, you don't want to get so rigid that you feel trapped by your habits; but just a few things on autopilot can really take the pressure off making so many decisions about your health every day.

DON'T TRY TO BE PERFECT!

Perfection is never the goal when it comes to your health—it's all about balance. We're all plain old human beings who will never do everything right all the time. Getting caught up in trying to be perfect is definitely a stressful way of living! Embrace your humanness, and positive changes will come much easier to you.

BE FLEXIBLE

What works one day (or month or year) might not work the next. Life changes, your body changes, and even your preferences change over time. Go with the flow! Learn to listen to your body and adapt as needed. You don't have to conform to someone else's plan or ideas about life. It's all about what works for you.

LOVE YOUR BODY

This entire book is about nourishing your body on a metabolic level. But in order to do so, you really have to come to a place where you accept your body's imperfections and simply want the best for your body (and your health). Getting healthy won't make your body look like a photo-shopped image from a magazine, but it will bring more depth to how you experience life and better health with which to experience it all!

LIVE YOUR LIFE

Eating and living in a way that promotes a nourished metabolism is awesome, but don't ever let it get in the way of living a rich and full life. It's okay to travel the world and lose a little sleep along the way. It's okay to go to your best friend's birthday bash and just eat whatever's available without worrying if it's ideal. It's okay to deal with a traumatic life event that means some of your priorities get switched around for a while. These things are just part of life, and trying to be healthy should never hold you back from experiencing it in the best way possible.

Thank You!

THANK YOU SO MUCH FOR READING THIS BOOK! I can't tell you how much I appreciate that you took time out of your day to read what I've written. And I would absolutely love to hear what you have to say about it.

So if you have any thoughts or questions regarding this book, please don't hesitate to visit www.livingthenourishedlife.com and go to the Contact page to find the best way to reach me.

If you haven't already, please join me on Facebook and Pinterest if you'd like to stay in touch.

Thank you again for reading this book. I wish you all the best on your own journey to health and wellness!

» *Elizabeth*

Read More!

LIKE WHAT YOU'VE READ? Check out my other book: *Love Your Body: The Imperfect Girl's Guide to Positive Body Image!* Visit *livingthenourishedlife.com/books/ loveyourbody* to learn more.

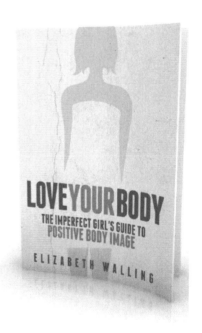

References

CHAPTER 1: WHY YOU NEED A NOURISHED METABOLISM

Barnes, Broda Otto. *Hypothyroidism: The Unsuspected Illness.* HarperCollins. 1976.

CHAPTER 2: STRESS: METABOLISM KILLER

Andrews RC, Herlihy O, Livingstone DEW, Andrew R, Walker BR. "Abnormal cortisol metabolism and tissue sensitivity to cortisol in patients with glucose intolerance." J Clin Endocrinol Metab. 2002.

Epel ES, McEwen B, Seeman T, et al. "Stress and body shape: Stress-induced cortisol secretion is consistently greater among women with central fat." Psychosom Med. 2000.

Whitworth JA, Brown MA, Kelly JJ, Williamson PM. "Mechanisms of cortisol-induced hypertension in humans." Steroids. 1995.

Raitiere MN. "Clinical evidence for thyroid dysfunction in patients with seasonal affective disorder." Psychoneuroendocrinology. 1992.

Cagnacci A, Soldani R, Yen SS. "Melatonin enhances cortisol levels in aged women: reversible by estrogens." J Pineal Res. 1997.

Carman JS, Post RM, Buswell R, Goodwin FK. "Negative effects of melatonin on depression." Am J Psychiatry. 1976.

CHAPTER 3: DIETS: THE ULTIMATE METABOLIC STRESSOR

Tomiyama AJ, Mann T, Vinas D, Hunger JM, Dejager J, Taylor SE. "Low calorie dieting increases cortisol." Psychosom Med. 2010.

Ross, Julia. *The Mood Cure*. 2003.

Mann, T. "Medicare's search for effective obesity treatments: Diets are not the answer." Am. Psychologist. 2007.

Priya Sumithran, Luke A. Prendergast, Elizabeth Delbridge, Katrina Purcell, Arthur Shulkes, Adamandia Kriketos, Joseph Proietto. "Long-Term Persistence of Hormonal Adaptations to Weight Loss." New England Journal of Medicine. 2011.

Jennifer S Savage, Lesa Hoffman, and Leann L Birch. "Dieting, restraint, and disinhibition predict women's weight change over 6 y." Am J Clin Nutr. 2009.

Lissner, L.; Odell, P.; D'Agostino, D.; and Stoke, J.; et al. "Variability of Body Weight and Health Outcomes in the Framingham Population." New England Journal of Medicine. 1994.

Guagnano MT, Pace-Palitti V, Carrabs C, Merlitti D, Sensi S: "Weight fluctuations could increase blood pressure in android obese women. Clinical Sciences (London)." 1999.

Faith, M. S., Scanlon, K. S., Birch, L. L., Francis, L. A. and Sherry, B. "Parent-Child Feeding Strategies and Their Relationships to Child Eating and Weight Status." Obesity Research. 2004.

CHAPTER 4: DIGESTION: THE ENERGY GATEWAY

Morelli L. "Postnatal development of intestinal microflora as influenced by infant nutrition." J Nutr. 2008.

H Okada, C Kuhn, H Feillet, and J-F Bach. "The 'hygiene hypothesis' for autoimmune and allergic diseases: an update." Clin Exp Immunol. 2010.

Sapolsky, Robert M. *Why Zebras Don't Get Ulcers.* Third Edition. Henry Holt and Co. 2004.

✓ Monastyrsky, Konstantin. "Fiber Menace: The Truth About the Leading Role of Fiber in Diet Failure, Constipation, Hemorrhoids, Irritable Bowel Syndrome, Ulcerative Colitis, Crohn's Disease, and Colon Cancer." Ageless Press. 2008.

✓ Torre M, Rodriguez AR, Saura-Calixto F. "Effects of dietary fiber and phytic acid on mineral availability." Crit Rev Food Sci Nutr. 1991.

✓ Van Immerseel F, Ducatelle R, De Vos M, Boon N, Van De Wiele T, Verbeke K, Rutgeerts P, Sas B, Louis P, Flint HJ. "Butyric acid-producing anaerobic bacteria as a novel probiotic treatment approach for inflammatory bowel disease." J Med Microbiol. 2010.

✓ J K Tobacman. "Review of harmful gastrointestinal effects of carrageenan in animal experiments. Environ Health Perspect." 2001.

Campbell-McBride, Natasha. "Gut and Psychology Syndrome: Natural Treatment for Autism, Dyspraxia, A.D.D., Dyslexia, A.D.H.D., Depression, Schizophrenia." Medinform Publishing. 2004.

Bruce Fife, Jon J. Kabara. *The Coconut Oil Miracle*. Penguin. 2004.

Kanauchi O, Iwanaga T, Mitsuyama K, Saiki T, Tsuruta O, Noguchi K, Toyonaga A. "Butyrate from bacterial fermentation of germinated barley foodstuff preserves intestinal barrier function in experimental colitis in the rat model." J Gastroenterol Hepatol. 1999.

Senthilkumar R, Viswanathan P, Nalini N. "Effect of glycine on oxidative stress in rats with alcohol induced liver injury." Pharmazie. 2004.

Zhong Z, Wheeler MD, Li X, Froh M, Schemmer P, Yin M, Bunzendaul H, Bradford B, Lemasters JJ. "L-Glycine: a novel antiinflammatory, immunomodulatory, and cytoprotective agent." Curr Opin Clin Nutr Metab Care. 2003.

Manco M, Putignani L, Bottazzo GF. "Gut microbiota, lipopolysaccharides, and innate immunity in the pathogenesis of obesity and cardiovascular risk." Endocr Rev. 2010.

Cani PD, Bibiloni R, Knauf C, Waget A, Neyrinck AM, Delzenne NM, Burcelin R. "Changes in gut microbiota control metabolic endotoxemia-induced inflammation in high-fat diet-induced obesity and diabetes in mice." Diabetes. 2008.

Robertson J, Brydon WG, Tadesse K, Wenham P, Walls A, Eastwood MA. "The effect of raw carrot on serum lipids and colon function." Am J Clin Nutr. 1979.

Cha TL, Qiu L, Chen CT, Wen Y, Hung MC. "Emodin down-regulates androgen receptor and inhibits prostate cancer cell growth." Cancer Res. 2005.

Wu Y, Tu X, Lin G, Xia H, Huang H, Wan J, Cheng Z, Liu M, Chen G, Zhang H, Fu J, Liu Q, Liu DX. "Emodin-mediated protection from acute myocardial infarction via inhibition of inflammation and apoptosis in local ischemic myocardium." Life Sci. 2007.

Okada H, Araga S, Takeshima T, Nakashima K. "Plasma lactic acid and pyruvic acid levels in migraine and tension-type headache. Headache. 1998.

CHAPTER 5: A BALANCED PLAN FOR EATING

Bisschop PH, et al. "Isocaloric carbohydrate deprivation induces protein catabolism despite a low T3-syndrome in healthy men." Clinical Endocrinology. 2001.

Liang, Jianfen; Han, Bei-Zhong; Nout, M.J. Robert; Hamer, Robert J. "Effects of soaking, germination and fermentation on phytic acid, total and in vitro soluble zinc in brown rice." Food Chemistry. 2008.

Salinas MY, Herrera CJ, Castillo MJ, Pérez HP. "Physicochemical changes in starch during corn alkaline-cooking in varieties with different kernel hardness." Arch Latinoam Nutr. 2003.

R. S. Mehta, et al. "High fish oil diet increases oxidative stress potential in mammary gland of spontaneously hypertensive rats." Clin. Exp. Pharmacol. Physiol. 1994.

Roberts CK, Sindhu KK. "Oxidative stress and metabolic syndrome." Life Sciences. 2009.

Raymond Peat Newsletter. "Unsaturated Vegetable Oils Toxic." 1996.

Bruce Fife, Jon J. Kabara. *The Coconut Oil Miracle.* Penguin. 2004.

Penny M. Kris-Etherton. "Trans-Fats and Coronary Heart Disease." Crit Rev Food Sci Nutr. 2010.

Slattery ML, Benson J, Ma KN, Schaffer D, Potter JD. "Trans-fatty acids and colon cancer." Nutr Cancer. 2001.

Chajès V, Thiébaut AC, Rotival M, Gauthier E, Maillard V, Boutron-Ruault MC, Joulin V, Lenoir GM, Clavel-Chapelon F. "Association between serum trans-monounsaturated fatty acids and breast cancer risk in the E3N-EPIC Study." Am J Epidemiol. 2008.

Yaemsiri S, Sen S, Tinker L, Rosamond W, Wassertheil-Smoller S, He K. "Trans fat, aspirin, and ischemic stroke in postmenopausal women." Ann Neurol. 2012.

Price, Weston A. *Nutrition and Physical Degeneration.* P.B. Hoeber. 1939.

M. H. J. Knapen, L. J. Schurgers, and C. Vermeer. "Vitamin K2 supplementation improves hip bone geometry and bone strength indices in postmenopausal women." Osteoporos Int. 2007.

Morley JE, Russell RM, Reed A, Carney EA, Hershman JM. "The interrelationship of thyroid hormones with vitamin A and zinc nutritional status in patients with chronic hepatic and gastrointestinal disorders." Am J Clin Nutr. 1981.

Semba RD. "Impact of vitamin A on immunity and infection in developing countries." In: Bendich A, Decklebaum RJ, eds. *Preventive Nutrition: The Comprehensive Guide for Health Professionals*. 2nd ed. Totowa: Humana Press Inc; 2001.

Van Immerseel F, Ducatelle R, De Vos M, Boon N, Van De Wiele T, Verbeke K, Rutgeerts P, Sas B, Louis P, Flint HJ. "Butyric acid-producing anaerobic bacteria as a novel probiotic treatment approach for inflammatory bowel disease." J Med Microbiol. 2010.

Kaunitz H, Dayrit CS. "Coconut oil consumption and coronary heart disease." *Philippine Journal of Internal Medicine*. 1992.

St-Onge MP, Jones PJ. "Greater rise in fat oxidation with medium-chain triglyceride consumption relative to long-chain triglyceride is associated with lower initial body weight and greater loss of subcutaneous adipose tissue." Int J Obes Relat Metab Disord. 2003.

Shari Lieberman, Mary G. Enig, and Professor Harry G. Preuss. *A Review of Monolaurin and Lauric Acid: Natural Virucidal and Bactericidal Agents. Alternative and Complementary Therapies.* 2006.

Fernandez ML. "Dietary cholesterol provided by eggs and plasma lipoproteins in healthy populations." Curr Opin Clin Nutr Metab Care. 2006.

Wheeler MD, Ikejema K, Mol Life Sci. Enomoto N, et al. "Glycine: a new anti-inflammatory immunonutrient." Cell Mol Life Sci. 1999.

Zhong Z, Wheeler MD, Li X, Froh M, Schemmer P, Yin M, Bunzendaul H, Bradford B, Lemasters JJ. "L-Glycine: a novel antiinflammatory, immunomodulatory, and cytoprotective agent." Curr Opin Clin Nutr Metab Care. 2003.

de Kooning JT, Duran M, Dorling L, et al. "Beneficial effects of L-serine and glycine in the management of seizures in 3-phosphoglycerate dehydrogenase deficiency." Ann Neurol. 1998.

Heresco-Levy U, Javitt DC, Ermilov M, et al. "Efficacy of high-dose glycine in the treatment of enduring negative symptoms of schizophrenia." Arch Gen Psychiatry. 1999.

Rose ML, Cattley RC, Dunn C, et al. "Dietary glycine prevents the development of liver tumors caused by the peroxisome proliferator WY-14," 643. Carcinogenesis. 1999.

Mauriz JL, Matilla B, Culebras JM, Gonzalez P, Gonzalez-Gallego J. "Dietary glycine inhibits activation of nuclear factor kappa B and prevents liver injury in hemorrhagic shock in the rat." Free Radic Biol Med. 2001.

Rose M.L.,Madren J, Bunzendahl H., and Thurman R.G. "Dietary glycine inhibits the growth of B16 melanoma tumors in mice." Carcinogenesis. 1999.

Gannon MC, Nuttall JA, Nuttall FQ. "The metabolic response to ingested glycine". Am J Clin Nutr. 2002.

Kaayla T. Daniel. *The Whole Soy Story: The Dark Side of America's Favorite Health Food.* New Trends Pub. 2005.

J. J. Rackis, M. R. Gumbmann, I. E. Liener. "The USDA trypsin inhibitor study. I. Background, objectives, and procedural details. Plant Foods for Human Nutrition." 1985.

Hiroyuki Kojima, Eiji Katsura, Shinji Takeuchi, Kazuhito Niiyama, and Kunihiko Kobayashi. "Screening for estrogen and androgen receptor activities in 200 pesticides by in vitro reporter gene assays using Chinese hamster ovary cells." Environ Health Perspect. 2004.

CHAPTER 6: SALT, SUGAR AND WATER MYTHS

Wormer, Eberhard J. "A taste for salt in the history of medicine. Science Tribune." 1999.

Dinicolantonio JJ, Pasquale PD, Taylor RS, Hackam DG. "Low sodium versus normal sodium diets in systolic heart failure: systematic review and meta-analysis." Heart. 2013.

Paul K. Whelton, MB, MD, MSc. *Urinary Sodium and Cardiovascular Disease Risk Informing Guidelines for Sodium Consumption.* JAMA. 2011.

Garg R, Williams GH, Hurwitz S, Brown NJ, Hopkins PN, Adler GK. "Low-salt diet increases insulin resistance in healthy subjects." Metabolism. 2011.

Bryant KR, Rothwell NJ, Stock MJ. "Influence of sodium intake on thermogenesis and brown adipose tissue in the rat. Int J Obes. 1984.

Krause EG, de Kloet AD, Flak JN, Smeltzer MD, Solomon MB, Evanson NK, Woods SC, Sakai RR, Herman JP. "Hydration state controls stress responsiveness and social behavior." J Neurosci. 2011.

Dulloo AG, Eisa OA, Miller DS, Yudkin J. "A comparative study of the effects of white sugar, unrefined sugar and starch on the efficiency of food utilization and thermogenesis." Am J Clin Nutr. 1985.

Hill JO, Prentice AM. "Sugar and body weight regulation." Am J Clin Nutr. 1995.

Meyer BJ, van der Merwe M, Du Plessis DG, de Bruin EJ, Meyer AC. "Some physiological effects of a mainly fruit diet in man." S Afr Med J. 1971.

Peat, Raymond. "Water: swelling, tension, pain, fatigue, aging." Ray Peat Newsletter. 2008.

CHAPTER 7: SUPPLEMENTS VERSUS SUPERFOODS

Zittermann, A. "Effects of vitamin K on calcium and bone metabolism." Curr Opin Clin Nutr Metab Care. 2001.

Gast GC, de Roos NM, Sluijs I, Bots ML, Beulens JW, Geleijnse JM, Witteman JC, Grobbee DE, Peeters PH, van der Schouw YT. "A high menaquinone intake reduces the incidence of coronary heart disease." Nutr Metab Cardiovasc Dis. 2009.

CHAPTER 8: HOW BETTER SLEEP CAN NOURISH YOUR METABOLISM

Leproult R, Copinschi G, Buxton O, Van Cauter E. "Sleep loss results in an elevation of cortisol levels the next evening." Sleep. 1997.

E. Donga, M. van Dijk, J. G. van Dijk, N. R. Biermasz, G. J. Lammers, K. W. van Kralingen, E. P. M. Corssmit, J. A. Romijn. "A Single Night of Partial Sleep Deprivation Induces Insulin Resistance in Multiple Metabolic Pathways in Healthy Subjects." Journal of Clinical Endocrinology & Metabolism. 2010.

Touma C, Pannain S. "Does lack of sleep cause diabetes?" Cleve Clin J Med. 2011.

Ferrie JE, Shipley MJ, Akbaraly TN, Marmot MG, Kivimäki M, Singh-Manoux A. "Change in sleep duration and cognitive function: findings from the Whitehall II Study." Sleep. 2011.

Dinges, D. et al., "Cumulative Sleepiness, Mood Disturbance, and Psychomotor Vigilance Decrements During a Week of Sleep Restricted to 4–5 Hours Per Night." Sleep. 1997.

Nofzinger, E., "Functional Neuroimaging of Sleep." Seminars in Sleep Neurology. 2005.

Ruiter M, et al. "Short sleep predicts stroke symptoms in persons of normal weight." APSS. 2012.

CHAPTER 9: SMART AND BALANCED EXERCISE

J. Henson, T. Yates, S. J. H. Biddle, C. L. Edwardson, K. Khunti, E. G. Wilmot, L. J. Gray, T. Gorely, M. A. Nimmo, M. J. Davies. "Associations of objectively measured sedentary behaviour and physical activity with markers of cardiometabolic health." 2013.

James H. O'Keefe et al. "Potential Adverse Cardiovascular Effects From Excessive Endurance Exercise." Mayo Clinic Proceedings. 2012.

Otto Mayer, Jr, Jaroslav Šimon, Jan Filipovský, Markéta Plášková, Richard PiknerOtto Mayer, Jr, Jaroslav Šimon, Jan Filipovský, Markéta Plášková, Richard Pikner. "Hypothyroidism in coronary heart disease and its relation to selected risk factors." Vasc Health Risk Manag. 2006.

R W Fry, J R Grove, A R Morton, P M Zeroni, S Gaudieri, D Keast. "Psychological and immunological correlates of acute overtraining." Br J Sports Med. 1994.

Park BJ, Tsunetsugu Y, Kasetani T, Kagawa T, Miyazaki Y. "The physiological effects of Shinrin-yoku (taking in the forest atmosphere or forest bathing): evidence from field experiments in 24 forests across Japan." Environ Health Prev Med. 2010.

Gibala MJ, Little JP, Macdonald MJ, Hawley JA. "Physiological adaptations to low-volume, high-intensity interval training in health and disease." J Physiol. 2012.

Hood MS, Little JP, Tarnopolsky MA, Myslik F, Gibala MJ. "Low-volume interval training improves muscle oxidative capacity in sedentary adults." Med Sci Sports Exerc. 2011.

Trapp EG, Chisholm DJ, Freund J, Boutcher SH. "The effects of high-intensity intermittent exercise training on fat loss and fasting insulin levels of young women." Int J Obes (Lond). 2008.

Cuff DJ, Meneilly GS, Martin A, Ignaszewski A, Tildesley HD, Frohlich JJ. "Effective exercise modality to reduce insulin resistance in women with type 2 diabetes." Diabetes Care. 2003.

Layne JE, Nelson ME. Nutrition, Exercise Physiology and Sarcopenia Laboratory, Jean Mayer. "USDA Human Nutrition Research Center on Aging," Tufts University, Boston, MA 02111, USA. Medicine and Science in Sports and Exercise. 1999.

Anderson-Hanley, C., Nimon, J.P., and Westen, S.C. "Cognitive health benefits of strengthening exercise for community-dwelling older adults." Journal of Clinical and Experimental Neuropsychology. 2010.

Chang YK, Etnier JL. "Exploring the dose-response relationship between resistance exercise intensity and cognitive function." J Sport Exerc Psychol. 2009.

O'Connor, P.J., Herring, M.P. and Carvalho, A. "Mental health benefits of strength training in adults." American Journal of Lifestyle Medicine. 2010.

CHAPTER 11: METABOLISM AND WEIGHT

Gaesser GA, Angadi SS, Sawyer BJ. "Exercise and diet, independent of weight loss, improve cardiometabolic risk profile in overweight and obese individuals." Phys Sportsmed. 2011.

Bacon L, Aphramor L. "Weight science: evaluating the evidence for a paradigm shift." Nutr J. 2011.

Made in the USA
San Bernardino, CA
02 May 2015